ROOTED

HOW I STAY *SMALL TOWN STRONG*
WHEN LIFE GETS HARD
AND HOW YOU CAN TOO

A Guide to Finding Joy, Learning from Struggle,
and Coming Together One Season at a Time

LEWELLYN MELNYK

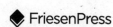 FriesenPress

One Printers Way
Altona, MB R0G 0B0
Canada

www.friesenpress.com

ISBN
978-1-03-9166077-3 (Hardcover)
978-1-03-916606-6 (Paperback)
978-1-03-916608-0 (eBook)

1. *SELF-HELP, DEPRESSION*

Distributed to the trade by The Ingram Book Company

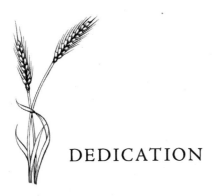

DEDICATION

This book is dedicated to all the small-town folk who have hidden scars, to all the farm families who continually make sacrifices to feed the world, and to those of you who didn't grow up playing in the dirt but continue to seek a better understanding of where your food comes from and the people who grow and raise it.

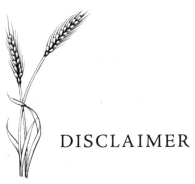

DISCLAIMER

This book is not meant to serve as medical advice for anyone suffering from depression, anxiety, or any other mental illness. While I reference medical studies and gather advice from mental health experts, this book is simply a collection of what worked for me and others. Everyone has a different situation, and if you require medical attention, please seek it.

TABLE OF CONTENTS

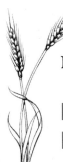

NOTE TO READERS

How to Face the World When You Don't Feel Like It (Turn up the Music)

"When I was looking for the words, somebody said it first like they knew me," sings country artist Maren Morris on "A Song for Everything," she wrote alongside Jimmy Robbins and Laura Veltz.[1] Do you ever feel a certain way but describing it feels impossible? Do you ever hear a song, and it perfectly describes what you are going through? Songs have been a source of comfort. They have even given me the strength to put one foot in front of the other on the hardest days. I don't just listen to music for entertainment. I listen to it for celebration, grief, and healing. I listen to it with my soul. Music has become a spiritual experience for me. That's because I've known what it is like to sit in darkness, in grief, in sadness, and continue to put on a happy face. In the moments when I felt happy, I could put on an upbeat positive song and dance around, or in the grips of a breakup, I could turn to a sad song while crying my eyes out. When I couldn't reach out for help, or tell someone I was hurting, I could always just press play and choose a song where someone was not only able to share those same feelings but sing it with the same raw emotions I was experiencing. It felt like justification. It felt like validation, even in my darkest days when I felt gagged by my depression. I know what it is like to say, "I'm fine," while wishing a quick end to my life. This was me at twelve years old.

In the nineties, many farm families were on the mend from the eighties' farming crisis and while the economy was starting to rebound, the damage on those families' mental health lingered, especially in small farming communities like the one where I grew up. Depression and suicide on farms and ranches are sadly common problems that have continued to exist. Farmers are at higher risk of suicide than other occupations according to a study that looked at existing data from the United States' National Violent Death Reporting System (NVDRS), including 140,523 farming- or non-farming-related suicides between 2003 and 2016 from across forty states.[2] A 2020 survey of Canadian farmers found similar mental health struggles in the industry. The University of Guelph study found that 45% of survey respondents had high stress, 58% were classified with varying levels of anxiety, and 35% with depression. In addition, women seemed to suffer more than men according to the data.[3]

Life on the farm is perceived as one that holds no space for weakness or vulnerability, yet I can list a hundred country songs that tell the story of hardships, heartbreak, and every emotion in between and I'm guessing most farmers will turn up the radio when they come on because they can relate to the lyrics. When I refer to farmer in these pages, understand that I mean men or women. And when I refer to women, I mean any woman who may or may not live on a farm, who may work on the farm, or works off the farm, drives a tractor, or doesn't drive a tractor. Whether your role on the farm involves physical labour or involves paperwork, meal preparations, raising future farmers, or you support the farm with an off-farm income, you are a farmer. If your role is to meet the needs of the farm and your farm family in one way or all ways, you are and always will be a farmer and I will refer to you as such in these pages.

Now that I've straightened that out, let's get back to the music, and the songs that most farmers are sure to relate to. "Jolene" by Dolly Parton, "Hard Workin' Man" by Brooks and Dunn (feel free to sing along using woman), or "Where Corn Don't Grow" by Travis Tritt are just a few tunes that people can relate to when talking about cheating, working hard, barely getting by, and hard times both on and off the farm. "Strawberry Wine" by Deanna Carter is sure to make you think of your first love, while Miranda Lambert's "The House that Built Me" might make you think of your first childhood home—this one gets me every single time as my childhood home has now been replaced with a new one. These lyrics might invoke strong emotions in the listeners, and they may even sing along with the lyrics, but some of those listeners often have an inability to speak candidly about their own experiences. Songwriter Lainey Wilson spoke about the best formula for writing a good song in an interview for Songwriter Universe. "I think it's important to tell the truth," she says. "For me, the songs that have changed my life, or songs that make me feel something, are the ones where people are being brutally honest."[4] Her debut album title perfectly describes her intentions: Sayin' What I'm Thinkin'. While we might not always be able to speak openly about how we are feeling, or say what we are thinking, songs can help us bring emotions to life. For me, they have made my life experiences seem more common, relatable, and somehow more manageable.

I hope this book will be that song for you. I hope I can help put words together that you can relate to your own life. I hope my willingness to share the struggles I've endured will help you know that feeling them and talking about them is something we should all do. As a kid, I often felt guilty for feeling a certain way and sat silent at the dinner table, struggling in silence with a notion that my problems weren't important enough to discuss. I'm clearing my throat now. I'm speaking up for you to know that it's OK to speak up. Not only is it OK, but it is essential for your well-being at any age.

I hope this book shines new light on the way you view your own mental health, whether you live in a small town or a city. Pain is pain and struggle is struggle. We all deal with hard things whether we are on a gravel road, a stretch of pavement, or a busy city street but we also have the capacity to lean into joy at every turn. I hope you take away valuable tools from this book to help you validate your emotions, practice compassion, and choose joy over fear every chance you get—kind of like the way I would choose dancing on a dirt road over almost anything. Choosing joy is my jam, and so is dancing with a good two-stepping partner!

I'm sharing the lessons I've learned while battling depression, anxiety, the pressures of being a mom, a wife, and a female farmer who has quickly become more outspoken than most in my industry. I wish someone would have shared these things with me when I was struggling in a job that I loved because I didn't take time for myself, when the pressure of becoming a mom would fill me with anxiety, and especially for those of you, who like me, have been in the depths of darkness and contemplated suicide. This book isn't meant as a remedy for depression. Talk to your doctor or health care provider if you are experiencing any mental health struggles. This book is meant only as a reassuring hand on your shoulder. These words are meant as encouragement so you can blaze your own trail after hearing about the path that I took.

Whatever part of the journey you are on, I hope my story will propel you forward in living a life you choose to live each day in the best way possible and help you get through the bad ones knowing there are better ones ahead. I hope what I share will keep you getting up every morning, excited to see the sun, and motivate you every day to do your best and be your best, and most importantly, to feel your best.

But I also know that some days you will barely feel like getting out of bed, and

I'm here to tell you getting through what seems like unbearable circumstances is possible too. This isn't a form of toxic positivity where I will teach you to only see the good with blinders on to everything else or that choosing to be positive will turn your life around. I want to teach you to see reality, deal with the bad or not-so-nice stuff, and recognize the good stuff, the stuff that is right for you, and move forward, confident in each step you take.

What follows are life experiences of overcoming depression as a child, managing anxiety as a young journalist and then again on the farm, battles lost (accepting that I am and always will be an overachiever), battles won (embracing that desire while balancing self-care), personal growth, and learning (lots and lots of learning).

This book is the result of a love of writing, a desire to be better, and also a longing to help others through teaching about mental health while healing my own hurt. It is my hope that as you read this book, the struggles we all feel from time to time won't feel so much like struggles at all. They are, after all, what makes us human and ensures we are there for each other when we need support. I hope being as painfully real (and sometimes funny, to balance it out) will help you turn your struggles into your strengths.

In these pages, you will also find music. I have found it to be such a comfort, an inspiration, and a get-moving motivator and hope that you will, too. Music has helped me to make sense of the world. Highly sensitive and empathetic people listen and feel music more intensely. Do you ever get chills when you are listening to music? That's caused by a release of dopamine in your brain. That release of dopamine can create feelings of pleasure and reward, which can lead you to act in ways that boost your mood. With music, this is a healthy boost! When you see a reference to a certain song, I encourage you to find that song on whatever streaming service you use and sit and listen to it, either as you read or when you get to the end of a chapter. Engage in the emotions that you feel when you hear the songs. What does it make you think about and how does it make you feel? Music acts like a time machine for me. Hearing Paul Brandt's *"When You Call My Name"* transports me back to a time when my husband and I attended Dauphin's Countryfest—an outdoor music festival we attended when we first started dating. The singer's band didn't get to the show on time to join him. My husband and I stood in the front row, his arms wrapped around me, listening to Brandt play this ballad with only his guitar and two other musicians who volunteered to play drums and piano for accompaniment. "I hear the sweetest sound, my world stops turning round, like

I'm on holy ground, when you call my name,"[5] the quintessential Canadian artist sang. Just hearing the first few notes of the song can make the hair stand up on the back of my neck. It is *our* song. It is the song we danced to at our wedding a few years after that concert and it will forever transport me back to that time where we both found new love. Meanwhile, hearing anything by the band Soundgarden will take me to a place of darkness, reminding me of a time when life was not so precious for me. As it turns out, front man Chris Cornell felt the same way, hanging himself in 2017. Not every song in these pages will conjure the same emotions for you, but I hope they will help you feel something. Music is my medicine. Whether it helped me laugh, or cry, it has always helped me feel. It turns out that honouring my emotions has been the best medicine for my mental health. I hope the music listed in these pages will do the same for you.

Some songs will be fun, some will be silly, but some might be hard for you to sit with. It isn't often that books come with soundtracks, but this one does. So settle down with your book and a set of headphones or a speaker and let's take this journey together. I'll hold your hand the whole way! I promise.

CUE "A SONG FOR EVERYTHING" BY MAREN MORRIS

To download the complete *Rooted* playlist on Spotify, scan the QR code
and hit play on each song when prompted during the chapters ahead, or cue up
each song on whatever streaming service you prefer.

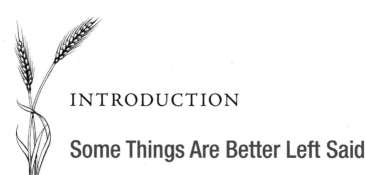

INTRODUCTION

Some Things Are Better Left Said

Lots of people have told me that some things are better left unsaid. Maybe for some people that might feel right, but for me, I think it is better when I say them. That's why I decided to share my story with honesty and vulnerability. While being vulnerable can be hard, it can also let others know they are not alone. Hearing other people's stories have been helpful for me. Since bettering my mental health has become my top priority, I've learnt that shining light on dark subjects takes away the sting, the hurt, and the shame that is often associated with them and makes way for healing.

Too often our small or rural communities have felt the hurt and experienced the grief of losing a loved one to suicide. I lost a childhood friend to mental illness a few years ago. The sting of that loss has stayed with me and brings back the loss as if it was yesterday when I hear of yet another farmer who committed suicide, or recently of a new mom and small-town teacher who suffered postpartum depression. Her only way to feel better, she thought, was on the other side of a gun. Small town living can be such a beautiful thing, but there are also struggles that exist here that are in the fabric of the lifestyle. It is those things I set out to talk about with this book, through my eyes and the eyes of others who also believe that some things are better left said.

COVID Crisis or Mental Health Crisis?

March 2020: All Manitoba schools are closed. The government announces that students will be homeschooled for the remainder of the school year.

I read the e-mail and choked back the lump in my throat at the news that I would be forced to teach my children at home. I didn't want to be a teacher. I never felt I had the patience to be one and definitely didn't have the training. I was scared. I was angry. I was overwhelmed before it even began. I wondered how I would manage my tasks on our grain farm while teaching my second and fourth grader. Seeding was always hectic on the farm, but this spring I would have to do all my regular tasks: making meals, picking stones, doing farm books, running back and forth to the field, all while teaching two kids full time. I remember sobbing on the phone to my friend Kathy. I walked out of the house so the kids wouldn't hear me crying. I stood on the deck and in between cries, I asked her, "How will we manage it all?"

I knew I wasn't alone. She also had a hand in running two businesses and held a council seat in the local rural municipality. I knew that Kathy and I, like so many other parents, were faced with the same circumstances because governments felt COVID-19 was too much of a threat to keep schools open.

For me though, I knew that being overwhelmed and overworked usually triggered my anxiety. I knew that I was in for another battle. One I had fought many times before. I knew that I needed to stay on top of it. It could be a real and serious threat to my mental health, and I knew I had to come out with both gloves on and swinging if I wanted to fight it. I had dealt with depression and anxiety before, so the circumstances made me angry about what was out of my control. But I was also prepared for what I was about to face. While I knew what I needed to do when times got tough, there were many people around the world who were about to walk into mental injury they hadn't experienced before.

When COVID-19 hit and people were in lockdown for months, something happened. Something happened that will forever change the way that people look at mental health. People who had never experienced mental health problems before suddenly discovered what it was like to have anxiety, depression, or both.

According to the CDC, only 11% of adults reported symptoms of anxiety or depression in January 2019, but over 41% reported having symptoms in 2021.[6] Mental health problems became just as big a threat to people's health as the virus itself. I watched it all go down. I watched it on the news and read the stories online. One night, I watched a news story about the isolation seniors were experiencing in nursing homes in Canada. Some of the seniors were isolated in their rooms for months without being able to go out or see family or friends. One resident who loved to go for walks explained to the reporter that she had no ability to see family or friends, no ability to get out of her room, and ultimately, she decided to exercise the right to die legislation we now have in Canada. She said that living in isolation was no way to live. It broke my heart to hear her story, but I understood it. I could see so many people, just like her, struggling with something that I had dealt with all my life. I heard a few months later that she exercised her right to die. I can't say I disagree with her decision given the circumstances. I have and always will fight for freedom of choice when it comes to women's rights, health care rights, and especially the right to die. Why should those decisions be anyone else's but our own?

I had debilitating depression as a child to a point where I gave no fucks about anything or anyone including myself. I also had anxiety as an adult that would take my breath away at times, steal my sleep, and cripple my body in muscle tension making daily tasks hard to manage. Hearing other people suffering with declining mental health broke my heart. The imposed isolation made me angry. It also broke my heart to see what kind of advice people were receiving. Some of the information was cringe worthy. One report recommended finding alternatives to face-to-face connections, while another said to stay off social media. If there was one time that we needed virtual connections, wasn't it during lockdowns?

I knew it was time to share my story. I had a realization that most people didn't have the knowledge I had about staying mentally well. I had learnt it out of sheer survival, through years of experimenting with what things worked for me and what didn't. I realized that I was heavily armed with so much knowledge and took on the task to write this book, documenting my stories for others. I am convinced that my story, and the story of other small-town women, would help to educate people on what mental wellness looks like, how to cultivate good mental health strategies, and how to do it under any circumstance. I knew, for certain, that I could help others so they wouldn't have to struggle the way I had in the past, and this book is the result.

I wish someone would have handed me this book years ago. The tools in here saved my life, but it took me decades to accumulate them all. Mental health is something we all experience. While mental illness can plague some people more than others, there is no quick fix for those who are suffering. It takes knowledge, self-awareness, good habits, and consistency to achieve mental wellness. I would be doing a disservice if I didn't share my knowledge. I would rather my long road be made a bit shorter for you. Maybe you struggle with mental health, and maybe you don't. However, I think the tips I share, along with my story and the stories of other women who have encountered hard times can help everyone through the tough times we inevitably all face at some point in our life.

It wasn't until recently that I could talk about my struggles with mental health. Just the thought of talking about my depression and anxiety held such shame and guilt that it would cripple me. But I know what it does when we don't talk about it. At twelve, I was supposed to be getting ready for church but instead, was concocting ways to kill myself. I held so much guilt in the way I was feeling that I was willing to take my own life rather than talk about how I was feeling. I know that sounds absurd, even now as I write this, but it is the truth. And my guess is that I'm not alone. Perhaps you were taught to hide your feelings, or never felt comfortable sharing them. Perhaps you felt ashamed to share them or were criticized when you did. Whatever your circumstances, you may find that you aren't being honest with yourself about how you are feeling. I know I am not alone in the struggle to give a voice to those feelings.

May this book serve as a guide on how to take care of your mental health and ultimately take care of yourself in the most meaningful way. I'm speaking up about mental health and sharing my own story to help you feel your best whether you consistently or occasionally struggle to feel well. After taking the journey myself, I am here to tell you that it is possible, even if you feel like you are in the depths of hell and can't find a way out. Maybe you've never experienced toxic thoughts before, but maybe you've had a Monday where the world felt like it was crashing down around you, or a period in your life that you felt flipped upside down, or perhaps when the whole world shut down because of a virus, it put you in a place mentally that you never experienced before. In those times of uncertainty and fear, there is a path to joy. I know, because I've walked it, ran it, or crawled down it, in pursuit of it. I'm willing to guide you there because I know how important joy is.

How to make yourself healthy and feel well is one of the most important tools you can learn. Nobody can do it for you. They can help you. They can guide you. But ultimately, you are here on this earth to look after your own body, mind, and soul. It's the most important job you will ever have. Sometimes that job is easy and doesn't take any maintenance at all. Other times, when you are feeling unwell or off balance, it is hard to identify what you need and why you need it. I can teach you. Let my experiences guide your own journey.

In March of 2020, while attending RISE, a personal development conference in Toronto, Ontario just days before that COVID lockdown took place, I made myself a goal at the end of the weekend that seemed almost impossible at first, but we all committed to leaving with a goal that we would work toward and achieve.

"Go all in!" we were told. Each one of us wrote something down in our fancy notebook we were given along with a roadmap on how to get there. We were also told to write it down in past tense, fooling our mind into believing that we already did this thing. Mine read:

I wrote a best-selling book on mental health.

I got home and decided it was time to start writing. This was the calling I had inside of me. RISE just lit the fire that was already burning. Little did I know, COVID would bombard those plans like a train wreck just a few days later. After homeschooling for a few months (and to be honest, even though I dreaded it, I did a damn good job), I took COVID as a sign to keep writing when I saw people struggling around me. COVID not only made this book possible, it also made it essential because mental health took centre stage. COVID made way for this message. I saw people struggling with isolation, lack of connection, poor exercise habits, and nutrition and recognized that many of them didn't have the tools they needed to nourish their mental health the way I had learned throughout my lifetime. I watched friends turn to bad habits like drinking or drugs to cope, and I knew it was time to start writing.

I hope my experiences and the advice I have gathered can teach you how to gain strength in your own life. If there is one thing I hope you get from this book, it is how to live a healthy and well-balanced life. And by healthy life I don't mean how you look. In fact, I hope you never equate those two things. Your appearance has little to do with your mental health. Your appearance is a by-product of your general health and well-being. I hope that you equate health with how you feel. And by the time you implement the tips and advice I have laid out in this book, you should notice a substantial difference in how you feel.

My hope is this book will make a difference for you. When you have a bad day, or a bad week, I want you to remember it isn't a bad life. Nothing is permanent, even though sometimes it might feel that way. There is a saying, "When it rains, it pours," and we know this one all too well on the farm, but there is also another saying that, "Every storm runs out of rain." Nothing lasts forever. Life is ultimately what we make it. And I'm going to tell you how to make it the best you can, not by pretending those bad days or bad seasons don't exist, but by acknowledging that they are going to occur and teaching you how to manage the bad days and lean into them as well as appreciate the good ones. I hope these tips will help you walk the road ahead knowing that you are not alone. We all walk the same road, some of us just have bigger mountains to climb and deeper valleys to crawl out of. But as long as you keep walking, and give yourself grace when you fall down, you will always find your way. I hope the walk becomes the enjoyable part. Falling down is a part of life. Getting back up is living.

I can use all the fancy metaphors in the world to paint a pretty picture of what dealing with a mental illness is, but it isn't pretty and it isn't supposed to be.

In the chapters ahead, you will see why mental wellness is important for everyone and why we should all make it a priority in our lives. You will also see what managing your mental wellness looks like in real life situations, through my own experiences and others. It is a constant ebb and flow, and some days you will feel hopeful and other days you will feel like throwing in the towel, but my hope is that you will take the lessons in this book and put them into practice in your life. Managing your mental wellness can be as basic as getting sleep, eating properly, and exercising. But it can also be a lot more than that too. Mental wellness can mean giving yourself grace, finding your unique identity, seeking connections, building confidence, validating emotions, and learning compassion. Mental wellness is the ability to manage emotions in a meaningful way that serves your body and your mind. Sometimes it is as easy as keeping a good routine, while other times it can feel like a fight.

CUE UP "FIGHT SONG" BY RACHEL PLATTEN

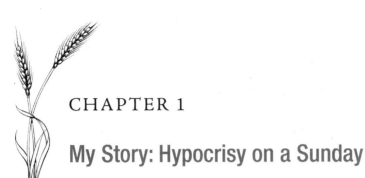

CHAPTER 1

My Story: Hypocrisy on a Sunday

It was a Sunday morning, and I didn't want to go to church. We attended the tiny United church that stood at the very end of Main Street in Inglis, Manitoba, population 930. It was the closest community to where my family farmed near Thunder Creek—a few miles east of the Assiniboine Valley and only minutes from the Manitoba-Saskatchewan border. Inglis is known for its prairie giants, a row of five grain elevators that have stood in that town since 1922. The church was small in comparison to the monuments of prairie pride but served as an escape and a sanctuary for farm families on Sundays. James Powell Laycock bought my family's farm in 1911. Four generations have since tilled the same ground and planted seeds there. The Manitoba dirt provided for us, as long as we had good weather, were willing to put in long hours of work, and make good decisions about what did and didn't make money on the farm. There were some animals on the farm over the years but my parents, Daryle and Veronica Laycock, focused solely on grain farming and had the belief that if we prayed to the good Lord, he would provide. I rolled my eyes at this idea. My mom was raised Catholic, my dad in the United church. I was baptized in the Catholic church, married in the United church, and have had my children baptized there as well, but I don't consider myself a good Christian in the sense that I don't have blind faith in the Lord. I never have. The only faith I've ever had was in myself and what I was capable of. I always held the belief that there was indeed a higher power, but I wasn't about to rely on him or her—and that's the way I saw it, even as a child.

Most Sundays our small prairie church with a huge spruce tree out front welcomed around two dozen members of the congregation. This particular Sunday morning, I was supposed to be getting ready for church like every other Sunday morning I knew before that, but I wasn't having it. I did not want to go. I felt, the only fulfilling things I got from church were the music, the lunch afterward where we drank super strong tea, ate raisin bread and sharp cheddar cheese, as well as the few minutes I got to play with a local farm family who had five energetic and kind girls. My mom was clearly fed up with my almost-teenage attitude this particular Sunday morning. She sat me down on my bed, in my basement bedroom of our 750-square-foot farm house that I shared with my sister, and asked me what was wrong. I thought about answering her, but I couldn't do it. I didn't want to go to church that Sunday because it felt wrong. It felt out of alignment with the way I was feeling inside. I had recently become obsessed and preoccupied with thinking of ways to kill myself and the thought of singing hymns and rejoicing in our church didn't seem to align with the emotions and thoughts I was having inside my head. I wanted, so badly, to end my life. I couldn't answer her when she asked what was wrong. All I could do was cry.

Not ready to leave my room without an answer, she sat beside me, looked in my eyes with this look of exhaustion that most parents have, and asked me again, "What is wrong, Lewellyn?" She kept pleading for me to tell her what was wrong. I knew I couldn't hide it anymore. I kept crying because I was also exhausted about thinking of all the ways I could kill myself. How could it be fast? What resources did I have available to me? How did I want others to find me when they came across my lifeless body? I was also crying because I felt guilty for having these thoughts. I was crying because nobody understood them. Crying because I felt alone and felt nobody could help me. Crying because my hurt was now causing other people to hurt and I could see it in my mom's eyes. I was crying because there was nothing left to do but cry. When I was sick as a little girl my mom used to rock me in her wood rocking chair while snuggling me with her pink corduroy nightgown. She couldn't do that now. When I was a toddler and couldn't fall asleep, she would sing a French lullaby to me called "Fais dodo" and rub my forehead. We were so far away from any sort of comfort like that now. She knew it and I knew it. Gone were the days where we would eat her homemade carrot soup with a slice of bread and cheese on the coffee table in our living room while watching *Sesame Street* together.

It felt like an eternity until I could muster up enough words to tell her what was going through my head now. I was so tired of listening to the same narrative over and over and trying to hide it in my actions and my words. I heard the words come out of my mouth as though it was someone else saying them. "I don't want to live anymore," I sobbed. That's all I got out and then I continued to cry, the tears were never-ending. Her response was to do the same, her tears now matching the flow of mine. I don't think she expected to hear what came out of my mouth that day. I don't think anything could have prepared her to be honest. And so, we sat on the bed, both exhausted, both in awe of what just happened, and both without answers of what to do next.

At that moment, sitting and crying with me was all I needed her to do. I needed her to walk through the pain with me. I knew she felt helpless when she began pleading again, asking me to tell her why I was feeling this way, but I couldn't. I could tell she was angry that I felt this way. She was confused, and so was I. I didn't know the cause or the reason why. But I knew I felt broken and guilty. So guilty. My parents had provided a good life for me, my brother, and my sister. We had a charmed upbringing with tea parties, gardening, kitties, bike rides, and we did it all with a backdrop of golden fields of wheat and breathtaking sunsets. They worked so hard for us. So damn hard.

My mom wanted to help me, but she didn't know how, and it was no fault of her own. She knew how to give us the best life possible as kids, making fresh bread once a week, teaching us how to dig in the dirt and grow the best garden, as well as how to care for others—including those little kittens we always had around the workshop. The age of twelve, when things got tough for me, was also an age when life got tough for her in an unimaginable way. Her own mother had died of cancer when she was the same age. I knew that even though she loved me immensely, she wasn't equipped with the tools to help me purely from her own life's circumstance. She made it to this stage in her life with all the resilience she could muster herself, learning to be a mother without one herself. At my age, I didn't have the emotional intelligence to tell her what I needed in those moments, and I'm not sure she had the capacity to hear them. I can tell you this was as hard on my mom as it was on me. I saw it in her eyes. I felt it. My dad, on the other hand, had the opinion that he should tuck and roll. Working hard on the farm allowed him to avoid tough conversations. He is the kind that would get up at 5:00 a.m. and go straight to work on the farm. He takes such pride in being a farmer, you can tell by the way he meticulously takes care of his farm equipment, how careful he is to watch his income and expenses, and the hours he spends to ensure a successful farm, even and especially at un-godly hours. At the time I was struggling, my dad was throwing himself into his work, doing all he could to provide for us, but in turn, was also doing a good job of avoiding my depression. To be honest, I was trying to avoid it too.

Our economic situation wasn't one that fostered good mental health strategies. I grew up in the eighties when the farm crisis was pinching out family farms from the landscape. Drought, high interest rates, and low commodity prices created a perfect agricultural storm. On March 28, 1982, just a month after I was born, *The New York Times* headline read: "U.S. Farmers Said to Face Worse Year Since 1930s."[7] It was no different in Canada where there were soaring numbers of bankruptcies and foreclosures on both sides of the border. I remember on more than one occasion, sitting in the office of the lender at our local credit union as my parents tried their best to find ways to keep their loans current. What happened to them, also happened to many other farmers across Canada and the United States. Many lenders called in loans, which meant they had the option to pay out what was left owing on the loan (many just couldn't do that) or be forced to accept a new higher interest rate, some near 20% —my parents at 24%. It crippled the daily operations of many farms who were lucky enough to not get foreclosed on like many others. My parents made the tough decision to carry on the family farm with the higher interest rates. My dad drove a blue Freightliner cab-over semi across the prairie to help pay the farm bills, and when we were old enough to look after ourselves, my mom got a government job in town to help keep us all clothed, fed, and made sure we always had new school supplies. But in the eighties and nineties when I was growing up, that tough economic situation meant sacrificing a new farm house my mom so badly wanted, so we could buy the equipment we needed for the farm. It meant we shopped at the local thrift shop for used clothes, and it meant we all helped grow a big garden. My mom would fix holes in pants on her sewing machine, can fruits and vegetables to save money, and almost everything we ate was homemade. It meant working hard. And then working harder. The poor economic situation on family farms didn't make time for self-care or rest, except for on Sundays when it was time to go to church—just like on the day I confessed my wishes to my mom.

From then on, both my mom and dad dealt with my depression very differently. Dad tagged out and became super focused on being a ruthless provider, while my mom became my warrior and advocate to find help. I knew my dad loved me, I never questioned that, but I knew that my mom understood on a deeper level what I was going through. And at a time of unknowns, and nothing short of horrific feelings I was experiencing, and no understanding of what to do about them, the sitting beside me was the saving I needed that Sunday. Even if she didn't know what to do, even if she was scared to death too, even if we both felt like we were on a sinking ship, she still sat there with me. Being a witness to my struggle was the only thing I required that day. And she sat there. I've learnt that nobody likes being around someone who is depressed, but the people who support you and care for you in those times are a special breed.

Now that I am a parent, I can understand what my parents must have felt. I'm sure they felt as though they didn't know what to do. I'm sure they also felt embarrassment and guilt, wondering how my depression would reflect on them as parents. Looking back, I had a lack of tools and resources to help me get better. So did my parents. They were not equipped to deal with my mental illness. Our small-town health care was meant for acute care. Hospitals were quick to fix a broken arm or cut head, but weren't equipped to mend broken hearts, or a young girl who felt depressed, alone, scared, misunderstood, and suicidal.

It was a tragedy for all of us. It has been tragic for many other families as well. It has been tragic that mental health services weren't available in our health care system for so many years, there were no mental health PR campaigns, and we are just now starting to see the conversation on mental health penetrate rural communities. There were no awareness campaigns about what to look for. There were no tips being shared on how to deal with depression. Even when my mom was asking anyone for help, there was not much available. There is now a better understanding of mental health in rural parts of Canada and the US but more education and strategies to combat mental health struggles and high suicide rates are required if we want our families and our communities to thrive, our rural communities especially, who are often silenced tragically with firearms or other means.

The cost of farming and ranching shouldn't be suicide.

My mom reached out and tried to find help wherever she could find it. That meant taking me to our family pediatrician, Dr. Elves, who we had seen since we were babies for everything from diaper rashes to allergies to yearly weight and height check-ins. I don't know what knowledge Dr. Elves had at his fingertips, but I remember the discussion we had. He said pick three things that really excite you or would make you happy. If you could do three things, what would it be? He was trying really hard to find something I could look forward to. I remember not being able to come up with anything. Nothing. I did not care about a single damn thing and I sure as hell didn't want to sit in a doctor's office talking about any of my desire or lack of desire for anything either. *I was broken. This confirmed it,* I thought.

He poked and prodded and offered suggestions, "How about going to Disney World? Would you want to do that?" "Sure," I replied. I appeased him. I had never been there. They say it is the happiest place on earth. *Maybe that could make me happy?* I thought. I also knew my family couldn't afford it and that was an elusive aspiration anyways, so I obliged. After an excruciating appointment where I would have rather been anywhere else in the world than in his office talking about my depression, his suggestion was to explore the possibility that my hormones were off- kilter. This was causing a chemical imbalance in my brain, we were told. He explained to my mom that I was growing so fast and my body and brain couldn't keep up. He prescribed the birth control pill to regulate my hormones. They agreed this was the first place to start.

Insert my period here. Open the flood gates, quite literally. I already had some spotting before this breakdown with my mother on my bed. But after taking the pill, my period really made its presence known. I had intense cramps and bleeding for two months straight. Again, we visited some other rather male doctors talking about rather female issues (let's take uncomfortable to the max). After some more poking and prodding in the most uncomfortable places, I was told to continue taking the pill as my period, hormones, and depression would work themselves out eventually.

I was definitely not sexually active at twelve. The pill was prescribed to regulate my hormones, regulate my period, and also alleviate my depression. It did regulate my period. It wasn't a magic pill. I took it every day for about fourteen years after that, coping, the best I knew how. Did it take the depression away? If you ask my mom, she says I was a changed girl. I don't remember feeling changed by any means, but I was finding my own path. I realized that if my mom was willing to do anything she could for me, I would do the same for her. I owed her that.

I think the doctor and my mom knew so little about how to help me at the time and they were trying whatever resources they had. I don't think it fixed me or changed me. I think it contributed to balancing my hormones which was just one piece of a much larger puzzle. A puzzle that would never be fully complete, always missing some pieces and forever changing its shape.

I was very self-aware, even at a young age, that I felt emotions stronger than most people around me. I would be the first to cry at a sad or happy part of a movie. I would be the first to fall in love in any relationship. I would even be labeled as that crazy ex-girlfriend because when I loved, I loved so strongly that I never wanted to let go, and I always wanted to talk things through when others didn't. I longed for connection and understanding. I felt as though people who really knew me were very lucky. I was loyal, empathetic, and protected other people's hearts the way that I wanted my own protected. I learned that my emotions were always magnified. If I was happy, I could feel it in my bones, throughout my body, feeling the sensations of relaxation and bliss throughout every inch of my being. But if I was sad, it was a deep, dark place that was hard to climb out of. It would consume me.

Growing up in a small town, many of us were not encouraged to talk about the hard stuff or took the time to. Farmers are a rare breed, the toughest breed around. Farm families, all across the Canadian prairies, had similar stories of experiencing overwhelming debt, inclement weather, and so much hard work. While farmers were always allowed to complain about the weather, it seemed they weren't allowed to complain about much more than that. Grain prices maybe, and perhaps whatever grader operators weren't grading the road properly. But feelings and emotions? Never. Farmers are a tough group to reach—both geographically and emotionally. They are tough. Tougher than most, but also unwilling to admit any vulnerability. If they did complain, someone would surely tell them to stop. I learnt that being small-town strong meant pushing through whatever emotions came up. After all, farmers could work for hours on end, day after day if they had to get a job done, and all because they were tasked with the ultimate job: feeding the world. Birthday cakes were often enjoyed during supper in the field. Nobody ever planned a wedding during seeding or harvest, because most people on the guest list likely wouldn't be able to come anyways. And if you had an emotional breakdown, it would have to wait until after the work was done, because there was usually rain, frost, or snow coming and there was no time to waste. Nature usually taught us to keep moving. There is also no end to work on the farm. It is an elusive goal that somehow, we think exists, but it is like chasing a rainbow.

CUE UP "FARMER" BY LEE BRICE

I grew up with the mentality that I had to be tough, but many times I knew for certain that I wasn't and I felt like something was wrong with me. I couldn't grasp the idea of putting emotions aside. It just didn't work for me. Why couldn't I bounce back like other people around me could? Why couldn't I just "suck it up?"

Why couldn't I "just get over it?" Why was I affected so strongly by some feelings and other people weren't? I was the super sensitive one in the crowd. I was the one with the big feelings. Whenever I heard someone say, "Stop crying," I heard in my head, *Stop feeling that emotion* you are experiencing. I would immediately tell myself to mask what I was feeling, and it always came with guilt for feeling it. The truth is, I was born this way: a super emotional, empathetic, and caring being.

Most of the feelings I had as a child were stifled by the urgency of almost everything on the farm, usually dictated by weather or finances, and it never allowed for much downtime or an opportunity to feel many emotions, let alone recognize them. The only times I remember feeling like I could relax and breathe as a child was when my family went camping in July. By then, the spring work was done, the crops were sprayed, and there were a few days to rest before the garden produce started coming in and harvest preparations began. Rest doesn't seem like the right word to use for camping because it involves packing up half the house to go live outside your home, sometimes without water or electricity, and most tasks, like making a meal or washing the dishes, took twice as long because you had to collect firewood, make a fire, or boil the water. The family time—away from the farm, the worries, and the unrelenting schedules though—was what could really fill an empty cup it seemed. It was a small window, and when it happened, it felt like winning the lottery. Some of my fondest memories as a child were because we camped as a family.

I believe I came out of the womb as an over-thinker and over-feeler. I'm quite convinced of it. I think my parents realized what a sensitive person I was and they tried their best to protect me from feeling too much when I was younger. We grew up with a Dalmatian named Bandit. The dog was living at our farm even before I was born. She was a permanent fixture until one day, I came home from school and she was gone. My parents had put down our family dog without telling me. I wasn't given a chance to say good-bye, to get one last hug. I remember being devastated. It was, in reality, just a life lesson. The dog was old and in pain and it was time for her to end her journey here on this earth. Her soul had outlived the body she was in. She couldn't even get up to go to the bathroom anymore. Even though it was the most humane thing to do for the dog, I was devastated that I wasn't given the opportunity to say good-bye. That, in itself, seemed inhumane to an emotional being like myself. Why wouldn't they allow me the luxury to even say good-bye? Perhaps, they thought, shielding me from those hard emotions was going to protect me? It didn't. It still hurt.

<hr>

CUE UP "EASY ON ME" BY ADELE

<hr>

I've since realized the best thing for my mental health is always feeling big emotions, sitting with them and processing them and never avoiding them. I grew up without validating many emotions. I hid my emotions for many years, trying to make them smaller on the outside even though they felt big on the inside. I hid them the best way I could.

It took years, in fact decades, to get to the place where I am now, a place where I am able to live my life in a way that honours my mental health. With the proper tools, I am convinced that I could have been here a lot faster, instead of spending so many years struggling. As a teenager, I turned to music (I sang, played piano and drums, and later learned guitar as an adult), journaling, focusing on friends and schoolwork, while holding down a part-time job. I was a people-pleaser and a perfectionist. Noticed how I said *was*? I've since learned that people-pleasing is a trauma response, but at the time, I tried to make everyone happy. Surely, if everyone was happy around me, I would be happy as well? If I could control my environment, which seemed to affect my emotions so much, I could control my happiness, I thought. I tried to make my teachers, my parents, my employer, and whoever was around me happy.

I worked hard at keeping everyone happy, and achieving big goals, all while continually distracting myself from my thoughts. I got my first off-farm job at thirteen, mostly because money was tight and if I wanted to ever own a pair of brand name *Silver* Jeans I knew I would have to pay for them with my own money. Plus, we were raised to work. So that's what I did. I would walk down to Main Street after school and start a shift at Russell Video, a convenience store with video rentals. When I was attending school at Major Pratt in Russell, I took on the role of co-president of the student council planning leadership conferences and spirit weeks for students, I got the highest mark in the province on the essay portion of our provincial English exam in Grade twelve (writing was a great outlet), and my friends and I were producing and distributing a high school newspaper once a week that included a portion that reviewed high school parties. It was fantastic for our readership but got shut down quickly by administration at the school. I was trying to do it all and please everyone and keep myself happy. It was immense pressure, and I couldn't sustain it. I countered the pressure of those things with going out, seeking connection with friends, which usually resulted in drinking, and ultimately a DUI charge when I was seventeen. I was figuring out this depression thing as I went. I had good days and I had bad days and I likely put a lot of grey hairs on my parents' heads while living under their roof. My parents would quickly realize that if I wanted to do something, there wasn't much talking me out of it. I was driven by emotion, and it would lead me almost anywhere I thought would bring happiness, and no one could stop me. No matter how much they wanted to protect me, no matter how much they wanted to shield me from painful emotions, they couldn't do it. No one could.

After singing the Chicks' "Wide Open Spaces" onstage at my high school graduation alongside two of my friends, I packed up and left to attend university. I remember my mom and dad standing on the front step, my dad had his arm around my mom, and she was sobbing. The kind of sobbing that says my last baby is leaving home—how did this happen? The empathetic emotional being who I was, I felt her pain and suddenly became an absolute puddle myself. As I drove off, my tears flowed, matching hers. Through my tears, I drove the three hours to my basement apartment, which was now a province away in the city of Regina, Saskatchewan. My tears kept flowing. This time, they were filled with fear and excitement for my own future. My mom and I likely had the same questions on our minds that day. How would I manage these emotions on my own? Where would my path lead? What choices would I make now that I was on my own? Spoiler alert: I'm thirty-nine and writing a book about why mental wellness is so important for all of us. I guess you could say I was emotionally driven to figure it out.

CUE "HOW CAN I HELP YOU SAY GOODBYE"
BY PATTY LOVELESS

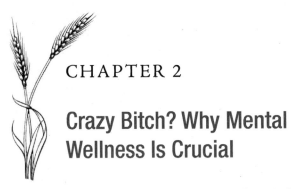

CHAPTER 2

Crazy Bitch? Why Mental Wellness Is Crucial

My experience with teenage depression isn't the end of my story. It is the beginning of a lifetime of managing my mental wellness. Does that make me a crazy bitch? Nope, it makes me human. I say "managing" my mental wellness because while wellness is my goal, I know it isn't achievable to be mentally well every day. Mental wellness is a spectrum, as some days you will feel amazing and mentally well and other days you might feel down in the dumps. Mental wellness should be a goal for all of us, but each day it will be different. Just because you have a bad day doesn't necessarily mean you have a mental illness; it just means you are having a bad day. My friend Whitney often says, "It is a bad day, not a bad life." She is right. We can't get hung up on one bad day. But if those bad days last for a long period of time, it might mean you have a mental illness. How do you know when you cross into that territory? The Mayo Clinic provides a long list of symptoms that may indicate a mental illness, naming withdrawal from friends and activities, extreme mood changes, detachment from reality, excessive fears, changes in eating habits, an inability to cope with everyday activities, and physical pain among many more.[8] The diagnosis is not an easy one and is never cut and dried. Mental wellness, on the other hand, refers to our psychological well-being. The Canadian Mental Health Association defines mental health as "a concept similar to 'physical health': it refers to a state of well-being. Mental health includes our emotions, feelings of connection to others, our thoughts and feelings, and being able to manage life's highs and lows."[9]

In my late twenties, I sat in the nearest emergency room in Russell (health care in rural areas here in Manitoba can sometimes mean a far drive to find help, but lucky for me, we have one within a half an hour from our home). I was unable to move my head or neck. If I forced my head any direction, piercing pains ran down the centre of my back. I had no range of motion and was as stiff as a statue. After being prescribed tranquilizers and muscle relaxants for a week, I could start moving my head again. In that moment, I had the realization that I hold stress and tension in my neck and jaw. I was not doing a good job managing my anxiety and stress, and the more I bottled it up, the tighter my muscles would get. They seemed to be a gauge of how I was feeling mentally, and at that time, they were getting tighter and tighter each day until I could no longer turn my head. I also became aware that I was clenching my teeth at night, holding my shoulders up around my ears, forgetting to breathe when I was feeling life's stressors, and staying too busy to take time to relax. The results were a trip to the emergency room and a lot of pain.

Sometimes, our bodies will tell us something is wrong before our mind even knows what is going on. There is truth to the saying, "You can worry yourself sick." Dr. Gabor Maté writes about the cost of hidden stress on our immune system in his book *When the Body Says No: The Cost of Hidden Stress*. "When we have been prevented from learning how to say no," he writes, "our bodies may end up saying it for us."[10] Learning to manage my tasks, thoughts, and emotions in a way that still prevents my body from saying no has been a learning curve. Maté writes about how many common diseases such as arthritis, cancer, diabetes, heart disease, irritable bowel syndrome, multiple sclerosis, and other autoimmune diseases may be prevented by exploring the link between mind and body.

I am more self-aware of my muscle tension now, stopping to stretch or do yoga when I feel my neck getting tight, relaxing my shoulders when they crawl up around my ears, or I am able to take a few deep breaths when I feel my breathing quicken or I find myself holding my breath. Mindfulness is just that, being self-aware of your body, breath, and mind. Comparing this kind of muscle tension to the way our brains work helps to describe what mental wellness is. If we keep going round and round with our thoughts, we end up tied up in knots, just like our muscles. Getting them untangled after an emergency room visit can take longer than being intentional in each moment and preventing it. Put a different way: you can't put out the fire if you keep feeding the flames.

So how do you identify what mental wellness is for you? I think it is different for everyone. Once you can visualize what you want it to be, it is easier to describe. For me, mental wellness looks like being productive and finding purpose, but not at the expense of my own health. It means being self aware while having the ability to calm my nervous system and regulate my emotions. It means satisfying my own needs, but being there for other people around me as well. It means sleeping well and having energy to get through the day. It means not worrying about everything, and not experiencing overwhelming fear, or feeling guilt about doing something or not doing something, or saying something, or not saying something. It means being confident in the decisions I make daily, but also realizing that I'm not perfect and giving myself a whole lotta grace. In short, mental wellness has to be personalized and everyone's definition will be different. As you can tell, I don't like sitting still for too long which sometimes comes at a cost.

CUE "SIT STILL, LOOK PRETTY" BY DAYA

This is pretty much my theme song here on the farm!

As I write this book, something I am deeply passionate about, I am careful to give myself a time frame to work on it. When I am uber-focused on a goal, I will put on blinders and forget to do anything else but reach that goal—in this case, write. Without discipline (and a whole bunch of other responsibilities here on the farm and with the fam), I could stay on my computer for hours working on this book. It may hit shelves a bit quicker, but if I am wound up tight, and an exhausted mess while doing it, the content in here won't be great for you as a reader. I will not have honoured my mental wellness either if I am not taking breaks to eat and rest. Instead, I make sure to take time for exercising before I write, take breaks to do farm chores, make time for family in between writing, and always stop for mealtime and when it is time for bed. I will admit, there have been a few really late nights and early mornings editing, but like I said, an important tool is the ability to give yourself grace in the process of achieving mental wellness.

What is mental wellness to you? It can be just as hard to define mental wellness as mental illness. It is unique to each person. For some people, it might mean identifying the things you don't want in your life. If you remove those things, what is left? Maybe you don't want to think about 432 things you need to do the next day while lying in bed at night. Or maybe you need a reason to get out of bed in the morning. Do you want to be more present when listening to your child tell you about their day when they get home from school? Do you want to go to work without feeling like you are dreading each day? Do you want your chest to feel like you aren't lying with 200 pounds of bricks on top of it? Do you want to slow everything down a little and stop rushing?

When our nervous system is jacked, our brains can feel like they are in overdrive. Remember when you were on a playground and someone yelled to you, "Think fast!" before throwing a ball at your face? That heightened sense of alarm can often take place in our brains. At Queen's University, Dr. Jordan Poppenk and master's student Julie Tseng found that an average person has 6200 thoughts per day. That means in one year, we can have over two million thoughts. Poppenk believes that mentation rate, or the rate at which someone's thoughts turn over or change, might have a link to the quality of someone's mental health and might help with early detection of schizophrenia and rapid thought in ADHD or mania.[11] I believe that he is just getting started in some interesting research about overthinkers like me. Think about when you are focused on one thing and are not distracted, doesn't your mind seem to work more seamlessly? When your mind is overwhelmed with thoughts, how does it affect your body or the way you are able to feel emotionally? Imagine trying to parallel park your vehicle while your kids are asking you a hard question from the backseat while your radio is loud. I'm guessing, if you are like me, that you may turn the radio down, tell the kids that you will answer them in a minute, and focus on what you are doing. If not, that parallel-parking job might end up with your pick up's rear end sticking out onto Main Street and you losing your cool. How does getting distracted make you feel? How does it make you feel when you have racing thoughts? If a thought comes in your head, are you able to manage it? If there are too many, do you become overwhelmed? Our thoughts can be distracting, similar to the radio or the kids in the backseat while you are trying to parallel park. Perhaps you are trying to write a test, and you keep thinking about what you have to do later in the day. Are you able to focus on the task at hand or do your future or past thoughts distract you? What about positive thoughts and negative thoughts?

Ideally, we would have a filing system in our brain, filing negative thoughts into the trash and positive thoughts would come to the front of our desk. We wouldn't think about the past or the future, just the present moment. But that's not usually the case. Author and motivational speaker Darci Lang believes we can train our brain to focus on positive thoughts and writes about it in her book *Focus on the 90%: One Simple Tool to Change the Way You View Your Life*.[12] While I think focusing on the positive has real cognitive benefits, I also think that too many thoughts and how we sort them can contribute to poor mental health. Being unable to sort thoughts is exactly what it is like living with ADHD also known as Attention

Deficit Hyperactivity Disorder. For people living with ADHD, there is no filing system. Thoughts swirl around until they are forgotten and remembered later, if at all and at inconvenient times, because that filing system doesn't exist. Whether you suffer from ADHD and have trouble sorting your thoughts, or just have too many thoughts that seem overwhelming, giving our brain a break, when it needs one, can be extremely beneficial to our concentration, our focus, and our emotions.

Do you ever have days when you have a to-do list in your brain that has twenty things on it and as another one pops into your thoughts, you redirect your thoughts to tackle it before you forget it? Now, you've lost focus of what you were actually doing and have one more thing added to the list. Where was I? See what I mean? Too many thoughts might leave us with an overflow. Perhaps that overflow is clogging up the system. Maybe we need a waiting room in our brain. Maybe thoughts need to take a number and wait their turn. Maybe we need to slow down the processing of all thoughts.

Shauna Shapiro talks about the effects that multitasking has on our brain in her book *Good Morning, I Love You*. She explains that when you try to talk on the phone and read an email at the same time, or switch back and forth, it is called spotlighting, and that constant jumping back and forth between tasks comes with a time cost. That cost is a rush of cortisol, bringing with it increased stress and fatigue.[13] This stress hormone, cortisol, is what weakens our immune system. That's why she explains that being present in the task at hand—and only one task at a time—is far more important to our mental health than the productivity, or lack thereof, of multitasking.

Another study by psychologists Matthew A. Killingsworth and Daniel T. Gilbert backs this up. It found that what makes us happy has far less to do with what we're doing and far more to do with whether or not we are present. The study suggests that a wandering mind is an unhappy mind. Their conclusion states that there is an emotional cost to having a wandering mind, one that thinks about the past or future instead of what is presently happening.[14] You might often hear people say you should live in the present, and this research explains why we should.

True mental wellness has to take into account that each day we not only have outside factors distracting us, but we also have these minds that wander. Throughout each day, we will deal with both thoughts that we perceive as positive ones and ones that we perceive as negative ones. Mental wellness isn't being happy and thinking positive all the time. While I think it is helpful to our mental health to focus on the positive, real mental wellness is the ability to manage all thoughts in a meaningful way and at a meaningful pace. When you realize your thoughts are racing, can you slow them down to a more manageable pace? Some people call this being self-aware. Some people call this mindfulness. There are so many definitions about what mindfulness really is. According to the magazine *Greater Good* from the University of California's Berkeley, mindfulness is "maintaining a moment-by-moment awareness of our thoughts, feelings, bodily sensations, and surrounding environment through a gentle nurturing lens."[15] That means being able to tune into sensing the present moment rather than thinking about the past or the future while observing your breath, body, thoughts, and feelings. Your focus should solely be on awareness and must be free of judgement. Simply put: perhaps thoughts aren't positive or negative at all; perhaps they are just thoughts.

Mindfulness is a learned behaviour and one that can be improved by things like affirmations, visualizations, and meditation. Mindfulness is one of the most effective tools to improve mental wellness, and I will talk more in depth about this in chapter 12. Mindfulness really encompasses what mental wellness is in simple terms: being self-aware and listening intently and carefully to our body.

Erica Hildebrand is a professional counsellor in Stonewall, Manitoba, who works with individuals who struggle with anxiety, conflict management, stress, grief, depression, and postpartum depression. In a personal interview about this subject, I asked her to define mental wellness. "Mental wellness is something that we have to face daily—dealing with the ups and downs of our well-being. We tend to think mental wellness focuses only on our minds and what our mindset is at the moment. But it's much more than that. It includes how we think, feel and act. It encompasses the whole of our emotional well-being when we focus on mental wellness."[16]

The Mayo Clinic's list of symptoms for mental illness can be things we experience often: being tired all the time, having low energy, or problems sleeping. Other things they name include mood changes, excessive fears or worries, or extreme feelings of guilt. Haven't we all had these at one point? I don't think that makes the entire population mentally ill. I do think it should make us aware that mental wellness is a range that changes for everyone, every day, and through different seasons in life. Sometimes it has a name or a diagnosis, but sometimes it doesn't. It can also show up in addictive behaviours like relying on substances to function daily, like alcohol or drugs. It might also present itself in gambling or risk taking.

It can mean having an eating disorder—either relying on food to make you feel a certain way, or restricting certain foods to make you feel a certain way. In other rare cases, like schizophrenia, it can mean experiencing hallucinations. The spectrum of mental wellness is one that we all experience, just in different ways.

What causes mental illness? While there is no concrete evidence, there are suggestions that a variety of factors may be to blame. Some believe that certain genes or traits might make someone more susceptible, while others believe it is a chemical imbalance in the brain. Other contributors may be prolonged environmental stressors (a pandemic, loss of a loved one, etc.) or inflammatory conditions.

There is no concrete evidence that one or another is correct, but perhaps, all of them have merit. That's why identifying a mental illness can be a difficult task and even more difficult, is finding treatments. I have explored treatment options, by researching through reading and trying different things, and I feel as close to an expert on the subject as I can get without a medical degree. I was taught in the school of hard knocks you could say. But I am not alone. In 2017, depression was the leading cause of disability according to the World Health Organization. Naming youth, postpartum women, and the elderly as three particularly vulnerable groups.[17]

In 2020, when the COVID-19 pandemic hit, mental illness ramped up to a whole new level. Researchers around the world are now realizing the implications that it had on deteriorating people's mental health. A report released in January 2021 named fifty long-term effects of COVID-19 that listed things like fatigue, headache, and insomnia for the participants. 80% of those who took part in the study listed at least one symptom.[18] The study showed the physical effects it had on people. But what couldn't be observed as easily were the results of isolation, restrictions, and the effect on participants' mental health. A headache and fatigue may in fact be a sign of deteriorating mental health. For example, a parent who had to stop working to homeschool their children experienced decreased income, additional family roles, and a decrease in self-care routines like going to the gym or going to get a haircut. The implications may show up "when the body says no," as Dr. Maté suggests.

With COVID restrictions present or not, everyone experiences times of isolation or a time when they have additional stressors in their life. But stress, itself, is not a mental illness. But stressors, over a long period of time, can cause a mental illness. The stressor itself is just that. It is an exterior factor. How you react to that stressor is an emotional response. That is why most of the stress in our lives is present because of how we process and react to things as opposed to the actual event itself. The tips and stories in this book will serve as mental health tools for your toolbox, helping you strive for mental wellness, teaching you some of the best ways to manage stressors, as well as the emotions attached to them, so you can tackle whatever ball is coming at you, and even if someone doesn't yell, "Heads up!" before it hits you.

I would argue one of the most stressful and hectic times on the farm is the time when fall closes in. The days get shorter, there are fewer daylight hours, the temperatures start getting colder, and we play a game with ourselves about how many days are left until the white stuff shows up. When snow and cold temperatures settle in, so many of the farm tasks get put to an abrupt end. Some years, you will get the equipment cleaned up and put away, some years you will get the garden veggies dug, and some years you will get the field work done before winter hits. Some years you won't. The thing is, we never actually know how much time we have. The season doesn't know what day of the calendar says it is fall or winter. It simply happens, and sometimes unexpectedly. That race we run to get all our nuts gathered before winter like the squirrels do can often be an excruciating time. It is a race, but you aren't sure how long you have or haven't before it is too late to do any more tasks. That unknown, the feeling of impending winter on its way, mixed with the long to-do lists, and the urgency to get it all done at all cost, can result in sheer exhaustion and ultimately poor mental health. If we aren't taking time to look after ourselves, in every day leading up to winter (and every day of the year no matter what urgency we may feel), we can reach the first day of snowfall and feel like we've been hit by a train. If we are intentional each day to look after our own needs, we can approach the change in seasons with the feeling that we did our best with the time we had but didn't sacrifice our mental health while doing it.

We know that we cannot eliminate stressors in our life, especially ones that are weather-related on the farm, but real mental wellness means managing stressors in a way that doesn't leave you feeling burnout, exhausted, sad, mad, or depleted. That management starts with managing our mind. As you'll soon learn, the connection between body and mind are more meaningful than any of us every imagined. Yomi Akinpelu wrote about the importance of self-talk in his book *Blow the Cap off Your Capability: Be Unstoppable*: "Your brain is like a supercomputer, and yourself-talk is the program that determines how it will run. Your mind is always eavesdropping on your selftalk."[19] In short, if you tell yourself you are not good enough, you will start to believe it. However, if you tell yourself you are worthy and capable of great things, you will become capable of great things if your thoughts lead you to actions.

Self-talk, or the feelings and thoughts we believe about ourselves, is crucial to how we operate on a daily basis. When you hear sayings like "Change the way you think and you can change your life," there is some truth there. It all starts with our brain but is tainted through our experiences. That's why throughout life, we need to learn resilience and gain confidence in our decisions, but also be mindful about why mental wellness should be the motivation for how we schedule our days. Stephen Covey, author of *The 7 Habits of Highly Effective People*, said it best: "The key is not to prioritize what's on your schedule, but to schedule your priorities."[20]

If you are struggling with a mental illness or simply want to improve your mental wellness on a daily basis, the steps I lay out for you in the chapters ahead will give you the knowledge you need to run that supercomputer the most efficient and most rewarding way possible. Taking care of your mental health, in simple terms, will help you to feel your best. Isn't that a priority we can all agree on?

CUE "CRAZY BITCH" BY BUCKCHERRY

Sidenote: I am not a crazy bitch, nor are you. We are just humans who require some grace. But this song is for fun so crank it up!

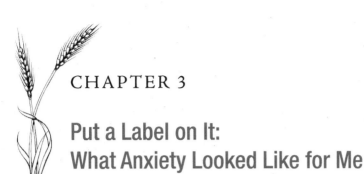

CHAPTER 3

Put a Label on It:
What Anxiety Looked Like for Me

If you are a parent, you know the feeling of getting brand-new school supplies ready for the kids to start school. There is something so satisfying about putting a new label on their shoes, clothes, backpacks, school supplies, and water bottles. Everything smells fresh and will never be as clean as the day that label goes on and they haul it off to school. Labels are great in this instance but putting a label on yourself can be very different. It can even be devastating if it holds negative connotations for you.

There are three kinds of reactions to getting a diagnosis from a doctor when it comes to mental health. The first is feeling relieved and happy to get a name for it. Like labeling it takes away the mystery of what it is that you are feeling. The label can now hold the blame: *It isn't me. It is the anxiety or depression talking.* This belief makes it easy to throw your hands up and relinquish control to the beast that now has a name. The second type of reaction when hearing a diagnosis for depression and anxiety can be *denial.* You may convince yourself that the doctor is wrong. Such a label is impossible to pinpoint, and no medical test can confirm such a thing. The third type of reaction is *acceptance.* After hearing a diagnosis, you are able to acknowledge the issue and engage in all the tools to tackle improving it.

I think the first two are the most common, especially in rural areas, because of the stigma attached with having a mental illness. I believe I went through both of these at different times. It has taken me many years to get to that third one, one of full acceptance and a passion for learning.

Let me tell you that the last one, *acceptance,* is the only one that serves your mental health and is the true path to feeling better.

My first label came in that doctor's office when I was a young girl dealing with thoughts of suicide. My label was *Depressed.* When I felt bad, I always just attributed it to my depression. I blamed it. It owned me for a long time. There was never a feeling of control over it. My second label came when I became a mom and both my babies were small. Denial and disbelief were things I turned to when I was diagnosed with *Anxiety*.

My daughter Ava was three and a half and my son Lane was just turning two. I welcomed motherhood in July 2010 just hours after being at a Dauphin's Countryfest for the day (nine-months-and-three-days pregnant) and following a good bumpy ride in the cab of a tractor while tilling the shelterbelt around our yard. I hoped bouncing in the tractor would bring on labour, but induction turned out to be the only way to turn this high-strung gal into a mother. For the next three and a half years, I took on the motherhood role while barely giving up much of my role on the farm, as I continued to do almost everything I was doing before our babies arrived. But it came at a cost. Farming is one profession where parents are tasked to do their jobs with kids in tow. It can be a blessing in many ways, but it is also a lot to handle when things get busy, which is why our family planning made sure the births of both our children didn't occur during seeding or harvest.

The winter of 2013–14, when I received my diagnosis, was one of the coldest I can remember. The weather would make it nearly impossible to take my babies to the grocery store. When you are a new mom who lives in the country, a trip to town to the grocery store is literally the best and worst thing you can imagine. Getting out of the house is glorious because it feels like absolute freedom. But packing diapers, wipes, snacks, toys, and other necessities for the trip takes a good half hour. Making sure everyone is ready, in a clean diaper, fed, and bundled up in winter wear and buckling into car seats is another good twenty minutes, and God forbid, someone filled their diaper after you have them dressed.

In those days, if I got to the store, it was an absolute miracle. I swear toddlers are trained in the womb about how to destroy the bottom shelf of a grocery store. Cans would start rolling down the aisle and I would try to keep my cool. Then one of the kids would get hungry mid-shopping trip and pick some grapes from the produce section and put them in their mouth. Or worse yet, they'd drop the one they plucked from the cooler shelf, it rolled on the dirty floor, and then they retrieved it and put it in their mouth.

It was hard to get everything on my list while having a little one or two in the cart as well. A car seat was too heavy to carry through the whole store, but when put inside the cart, there was no room left for groceries. If they weren't in car seats, they would fight to ride in the cart. Many times, I had retrieved bread, milk, and a couple of apples and suddenly there was no room left without piling items on top of someone. Were they better left to walk and destroy the aisles or better to be confined in the cart and take up the room meant for groceries? It was all too much. Any freedom I felt about leaving the house was replaced with trying to keep my cool and fighting back tears until I could get the kids back into the vehicle and head for home.

It was so cold that we could not go out for any kind of outing as the temperatures were deemed too dangerous to take two toddlers out of the house, so we hunkered down at home for the majority of our days. Short trips from the house to the truck were enough to take their breaths away and sting their little faces. The days seemed so long. My husband was taking care of our herd of cows, feeding them every day or two while still trying to haul out our grain to the elevator. He wasn't home much beyond eating and sleeping. Do you know what's even worse for a new mom than being at home with two babies all day and nobody to talk to? Being at home with two babies all day for days and days at a time and unable to leave your space (which at that time was a 700-square-foot house trailer). The demands of being a mom, the isolation and lack of connection, little sleep, and not great nutrition wound me up tighter than a yo-yo. I was in a bad place. I knew I needed a break. Something was about to give.

CUE UP "SMOKE BREAK" BY CARRIE UNDERWOOD

I would never have guessed that a break would have brought on my next diagnosis, but it did. In fact, it took a break for the adrenaline to stop flowing long enough that my body started screaming *no* while aboard a plane.

I asked my parents to take the kids for a few days, and my husband and I booked a trip to Jamaica. I remember booking it for only four nights and five days because how in the world could I be away from my babies for more than that? I couldn't wait to get a break, but the mom guilt was crippling. I felt such shame admitting I needed to get away from my kids. I had a great husband. I loved my kids and life was good. Wasn't it? I was grateful for what I had, but I was feeling so awful day after day. I felt awful with the very admission that I needed a break. I knew if I didn't take one, I wouldn't be able to continue momming as hard as I was. *What was wrong with me?* I thought.

I remember the vacation went by in a flash. I remember sitting on the beach and wishing time would just slow down. How did the days at home seem so long and here they were a fraction of the time? It was the first taste of real rest and relaxation I felt since my kids were born. Then, as quickly as it began, the vacation was over.

As the plane took off for our flight back to cold and snowy Manitoba, I began to feel my face go numb. First my teeth, then my mouth, and then most of my face. I was hot and lightheaded. Then I was passing out. But before I did, I managed to barely move my lips enough to whisper to my husband, "I really don't feel good. Something is very wrong." In a matter of minutes, flight attendants and doctors on board the plane came to my rescue, laying me down and checking my heart rate and pulse. The conclusion from people around me was I had a sunburn, got too hot on the plane, or I drank too much on holiday. When I got home, the symptoms followed me. They would wake me in the middle of the night and it felt like urgency for something but I didn't know what. My heart would be racing, I was hot, then shivering cold, I couldn't breathe, I felt like passing out again. These symptoms came over and over, night after night. It would wake me from my sleep and it felt horrific, like nothing I had experienced before.

When I visited the local clinic, they assured me they would check my heart and figure out why it was happening. They ran many tests, mostly looking at my heart. I was born with an irregular heartbeat, so perhaps that had something to do with it? But it didn't. All the tests came back normal. Meanwhile, I was still having symptoms. I remember sitting in the doctor's office alongside my husband and feeling so deflated and saying to the doctor, "What is it then?" His response felt like a slap in the face. "I think it is just anxiety." *Just anxiety?* I thought. What does that even mean? If he uses the word *just*, then I told myself it must not be a big deal. I was playing the denial game. I was denying the fact that this new label was crippling me. The doctor downplayed it, and so I felt I should, too.

I convinced myself it wasn't a big deal, but I knew it was. I was losing hours and hours of sleep night after night. I was exhausted and looking after two little humans who relied on me for everything. "What should I do?" I had asked him in the doctor's office. "Look online," he said. "There are lots of resources online."

So I did, Googling as much as I could about anxiety. I did learn that anxiety can manifest into a panic attack with the same symptoms as a heart attack: palpitations, pounding heart, sweating, trembling, shaking, chest pain, nausea, or abdominal distress. It can also be dizzy, unsteady, faint, lightheaded, chills or hot flashes, numbness, and tingling. He was right. My heart sank. I just got another label. Now, I had *Anxiety. Here I go again*, I thought.

I took whatever tips or tricks I could find and put them into practice: drink chamomile tea before bed, write in a journal, talk to a counsellor, and get exercise. I was so far down the anxiety hole I had dug myself already that I wasn't sure what was working and what wasn't and I just kept trying different things. Some things worked better for me than others, especially exercise. The exercise calmed my body, calmed my mind, and helped me sleep better. This was the first thing that I turned to that seemed to work the best and so I started relying on it to survive each day.

What started out as a survival skill for my anxiety turned into a love of running. If you would have asked my parents when I was born if they ever thought I would become a runner, I am convinced their answer would have been no. That's because I was born with congenital talipes equinovarus (CTE). Also known as clubfoot, the condition causes a baby's feet to turn inwards and downwards. Right after birth, my mother was assigned to the task of doing exercises with my legs and feet to try and get them to straighten out. After four weeks of trying, the doctors decided it was time to put casts on both my legs. After another few weeks of casting, I wore corrective shoes that were attached to each other with a straight metal bar, ensuring that my feet would straighten out enough so that I would be able to walk. And I did, but was forced to wear corrective shoes (pairs without bars thankfully) until the age of six. I could walk fine and appeared to be like any other kid in my class by the time I hit kindergarten. It was no longer an issue for me. I am thankful my parents took the precautions they did at such an early age as to save me from further problems in my future. The only sign of CTE I present now, thirty-nine years later, is a left foot that sometimes turns in when I am tired.

My love of running is the result of struggling with anxiety. Whenever I would wake up in the night with a panic attack, I would put on my winter clothes, and my winter boots, and head outside. I would walk in the dark, silent, cold night until my heart quit racing and I could breathe again. Then I would go back inside and crawl back into bed. I was coping. Day after day I did this. And I started feeling better. The panic attacks were coming less often, and I was able to go back to sleep faster. *Maybe there was something to this?* I thought. After all, I was willing to try anything. If exercise was working, then I would commit myself to daily exercise. I would have committed to anything at that point. That's just how awful I was feeling. I would go for a walk at night when I needed it and then added in one every morning. I then transitioned from walking to running.

When I first started, my husband would watch the kids, and I would run in my winter gear no matter how cold it was. I would even be running in my big black Sorel winter boots. They were so heavy. But when it is cold outside, and you live in rural Manitoba, and you need to run, that is just what you do. I did this day after day. At first, I would run from one hydro pole to the next, then walk one, then run one. Slowly, I gained endurance. Winter turned to spring and soon I would run two hydro poles and walk one. I traded in my winter boots for running shoes, which made running seem like a breeze now. By the time summer came, I could run a quarter of a mile without walking, then half a mile. I improved over time. I was feeling better. Maybe it was the thirty minutes out of the house alone that I needed, maybe it was the exercise, maybe it was the music in my headphones or the sunshine on my face, but whatever it was I wasn't going to change anything I was doing. I was finally feeling better and it was so worth it. I had some bad nights, don't get me wrong, but when I did, I made sure that the next morning I just ran harder and longer so I would sleep better the next night.

One day following my new routine, the mother of an Olympic curler sent me on my next mission. If you aren't familiar with curling, it is a very patriotic game here in Canada (right up there with hockey) where rocks are thrown down the ice, teammates sweep with brooms to control speed and how fast it curls, and the team with the closest rocks to the centre of the house (painted rings in the ice) score the points. In most small-town curling rinks, many people do this game with beverages close by. It is a game of socializing in small-town Manitoba during the winter months when bonspiels are some of the only community outings planned. In 2014, Jennifer Jones' rink was representing Canada at the Olympic level, and one of her teammates was a former co-worker of mine. I followed their journey closely. One morning, a reporter on CTV was interviewing Jones' parents, eventually turning to questions about the curler's raising. I remember Carol Jones talking about how Jennifer comes by her athletic skill naturally as Carol herself had become a marathon runner. She would go running to get out of the house and get a break from the kids, and eventually was so good at it and liked it so much, she ended up doing marathons. I connected with her story and it stayed with me. I decided I would run the five-kilometre race in Brandon's YMCA spring run. I trained the best I could by running a little farther each day using hydro poles along my gravel road as mini mile markers.

When race day came, I knew nothing about what was about to happen. We all lined up. The long- distance runners went first. The horn blew and off they went...first the group running twenty kilometres, then the people doing fifteen kilometres, then ten kilometres. Finally, it was my turn. The horn blew and off we went. I felt amazing. For the first time, I felt like a real-life, actual runner. People along the route were cheering for me. They were yelling, "Way to go!" or "You are doing so good—keep going!" I remember the tears running down my cheek. It was so emotional. These people were actually proud of me. Their support meant so much to me. Up until that point, my family and friends would ask me, "Why are you running?" I would say, "Because I feel better and I sleep better." They didn't really understand my anxiety. "You have to run just to feel better?" I couldn't explain just how crucial it was to me. It was, in many ways, my daily survival.

The strangers on the side of the race route didn't care why I was doing it, and they were all out there cheering for me anyways. They were all smiling and waving noisemakers, and I felt as though they were validating the fact that I had battled anxiety and I was winning. They could see it on my face and I could feel it with every stride. I crossed the finish line and I could see my husband and my kids waiting. The tears kept coming. I was in a full-blown ugly cry. (I'm really good at that by the way.) I felt like this race saved me. But really running was what saved me, so I could be the person, the wife, and mother I wanted to be. I realized I didn't need people cheering from the side of the road, but I did need to cheer for myself every step of the way. Their cheering felt really good, but my inside cheers were far more important.

I went on to run more five-kilometre races, some ten Ks, a fifteen K, a few twenty-kilometre races, and a couple of sprint duathlons.

It has been eight years since that first race, and now I schedule daily exercise to feel my best and achieve mental wellness. The physical wellness goes hand in hand with it as well. They are so connected I've learned. One of my favourite sayings is "Miles change you." There is truth in this saying. With each run I do, I know this to be true. They change you into a stronger person, physically, mentally, and emotionally.

For me it is running, but in the next chapter, we will see why exercising (in any way) is the most important thing you can do for brain health and mental wellness.

CUE "RUN" BY ONEREPUBLIC

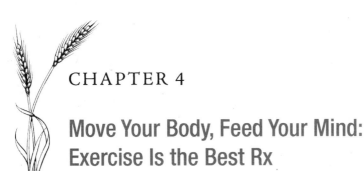

CHAPTER 4

Move Your Body, Feed Your Mind: Exercise Is the Best Rx

"You are only one workout away from a good mood." I don't know who said this first, but I assure you it is completely true and also the reason you will see it in almost every gym, workout space, trail, track or schoolyard. There is nothing better for your mental health than exercise.

I always thought when I was younger that I wasn't athletic. I loved biking and figure skating as a kid. I also really enjoyed playing baseball with my family. But when it came time to try out for all the varsity sports teams in high school, I never made the cut. I went to a school where you were either an athlete or you weren't. You either played the game, or you sat on the side and cheered for the Trojans (our high school team). I did my part. I cheered for the Trojans every single time. Not because I didn't want to play, but because I was never given the opportunity to play. I'd try out and never make the team. I learned from those experiences that I wasn't an athlete. That's what my brain heard. I wasn't meant to play sports, or so I thought.

My perspective changed when I got out of high school and rec teams and college sports welcomed anyone who wanted to play. I joined a curling league in college and loved it. Remember when I said the game of curling is also a game of socializing? I loved giggling down the ice as my teammates and I joked about how unathletic we really looked while sweeping the rock and trying not to land square on our tailbone on the ice. If you've ever done this, you know that it is all too common and the only thing that hurts worse than your tailbone is your pride when you are laid out flat on the cold, hard ice and the back of your head goes *smack*. Wipe-outs aside, curling was always so much fun with friends. I always enjoyed playing baseball too, so I joined a slow pitch recreation league when I was working as a reporter in Brandon with a team called the AgCatz. I loved it. My teammates were mostly working in the ag industry and I was in media, but being the farm kid that I was, we meshed perfectly. I was born and raised in agriculture. These were my people. I also joined a volleyball rec league as an adult, and again, filled a void that was missing in my younger years. I made some lifelong friends on both of those teams, and I really enjoyed playing, even though, my skillset was not at the same level as those who had played in high school. I didn't let that stop me. I was getting exercise, and it felt good to move my body and to play on teams with people who all supported one another. My brain was getting rewired to believe that I could play sports.

Even still, as a young adult, I didn't exercise that much. I did activities for fun like rollerblading. I didn't realize the importance of exercise to my mental health until that anxiety shit-storm of 2013 as a young mom.

Running brought such relief. I didn't need to run races. But running those races gave me a reason to run. It was a reason to train. I could set a goal and find a training plan that had tangible numbers attached to them. The races and the training schedules kept me accountable. Because I knew myself and how easy it would be to say I am not going to run today because I don't feel like it. So I kept myself accountable with running those races, at least one a year. I marked the distances I would run each day, laying out a sixteen-week training schedule at a time. I took the guess work out of it. I knew that on Monday, Wednesday, and Friday I would do a run. Tuesday and Thursday I would bike or some other kind of cross-training activity and that every Saturday I would do weights. Every Sunday was my yoga day. It made it really simple. I had a plan. I hung it on the fridge and would see it every day. I woke up and I would know what I had to do each morning. I was creating a habit. A routine that was the best thing for my mental health. Even when I am not training, I like to get my workout done in the morning because keeping a routine makes me accountable. I know it makes me feel better, so I schedule it in.

CUE "RUN" BY LAUREN ALAINA

Exercise releases feel-good endorphins. These are natural brain chemicals that can make us feel good after we have had some exercise. That boost in our mood is the single most important thing you can do to improve your mental wellness. Fitbit blog writer Amanda Williams covers the topic in "Five Exercises That Help Manage Anxiety—And One That You May Want to Avoid" where New York City clinical psychologist Ben Michaelis, PhD, weighs in, "The data on cardiovascular exercise and mental health is airtight," he says. "Patients I work with have to be doing some kind of exercise or they're not taking care of their mental health."[21] A study published in the *Journal of Sport and Exercise Psychology* asked people to rate their mood immediately after periods of physical activity. Researchers found that the participants felt more content, more awake, and calmer after being physically active compared to periods of inactivity.[22]

Exercise improves mental health because it boosts those endorphins, boosts your self-esteem, takes your mind off of your worries (because you are only focused on the task at hand), can help you get more social interaction in a group setting, and can provide a helpful coping mechanism for your mental wellness. That last one might be the most powerful. If you know you are exercising because it improves your mental health, you are more likely to do it.

Saying you are going to do it and actually doing it is where the mental strength comes in. And if you are already mentally unwell, just making the first move might be the hardest. But if someone told you that if you just ran around the block, then you would sleep better tonight, would you do it? If someone said if you biked to work today, you would not yell at your kids when you get home, would you do it? The reason why you exercise needs to be clear in your mind to motivate you to do it.

Let me be clear about this. The days when you feel the most unwell are the days you need to move your body the most. Don't let a bad mental health day be the reason you don't exercise. Let it be the reason you do.

Making time to get exercise in your life, if you haven't already, is no easy task. What does that look like if you are working, raising kids, and running to hockey or dance three times a week? It might look like getting up earlier to fit it in. It might mean doing it after you tuck kids into bed. It might mean pushing a stroller if you have nobody to watch your little ones. It might look like big winter boots, in the dead of winter, in the middle of the night, because you are having an anxiety attack. It doesn't always look pretty, and it doesn't always mean you are wearing some fabulous workout clothes with your hair pulled back and your makeup on.

I follow a lot of women (and some men) on my Instagram feed that are influencers in the health and exercise industry. I love all the inspiration I get and these pages absolutely give me benefit. They provide ideas for workouts, workout videos, and instruct on how to make a good training schedule. However, I absolutely hate that most of them will have a full face of makeup, their hair is curled, and they are lifting weights. Exercise does not look like this. It can be baggy clothes, bedhead, and sweat dripping down your face. Don't be intimidated by what you think you should look like when exercising. Just do the push-up and let your flab hang down. Celebrate the fact that you did it for your mental health, then by all means, go clean yourself up and do your hair and makeup.

I want you to know that it isn't about looking a certain way. It is about feeling a certain way.

When I first started working out, I did it in my pyjamas. I'm not even joking. I would roll out of bed, go downstairs with bedhead, and start working out in my pyjamas, because I knew that I had to do it before my kids woke up and if I didn't, I wouldn't do it. Sometimes, I do it in just a bra and shorts. Very rarely do I wear my prettiest workout clothes. It doesn't matter what you wear. It is that you are there. (I stole this quote from my mom who used to say this about church.) The message here is simply: doing the thing is more important than what you are wearing while doing it. What matters is that you do the exercise, even if it is in your pyjamas, or even in the middle of the night, or even when you would rather be doing anything else. Hear me when I say this. In fact, get your highlighter out, mark this page, write it in big letters on your fridge or on your bathroom mirror so you see it every morning: *Making time for exercise is the absolute most important thing you can do for your mental wellness.* Period. That's it. It is that simple.

Here is your reminder: You are only one good workout away from a good mood!

This is where I urge you to find something you like to do. You don't have to run, bike, or lift weights if you hate those things. But I do urge you to try a few things before you decide which option is a good fit for you. While running is my happy place and cardio will give you the most bang for your buck, I also enjoy doing Zumba. Zumba makes me super happy. We live smack dab in the middle of the prairies, but nothing brings me more joy than doing Zumba on a beach in Mexico (even more fun after a couple cocktails). I highly recommend it to anyone if you have the chance. If that's not your jazz, and you like a sport and can join a team, then do that. But also find something you can do on a regular basis. Consistency is the key when it comes to moving your body (and looking after your mental health). I can't do Zumba on a beach every day. I can do a Zumba workout video in my basement, so sometimes I will do that, but often it is running. One of the simplest things you can do is just lace up some shoes and go for a walk. Make sure to find something you can do every day that includes moving your body.

When I say cardio is going to give you the most bang for your buck, it really is true. Getting your heart rate up helps to stimulate parts of your brain that aren't as responsive when you're feeling depressed. It increases brain circulation and brain function. More blood to the brain means you are feeding your brain and helping it to work better. Maybe you have heard of a runner's high. This is when your brain releases those endorphins I mentioned earlier. These are neurotransmitters that stimulate the release of brain chemicals that help regulate your mood like dopamine, norepinephrine, and serotonin. It also helps regulate your body's stress hormones, such as adrenaline and cortisol.

Serotonin is the money maker here, so if you want to put money in the bank when it comes to boosting your mood, this is the one you want to make a deposit with. Ultimately, that's how you have to look at exercise: moving my body equates to feeling happier.

Exercise = Happy Brain = Happy Thoughts
Maybe you want to write that on your mirror too?

Get the point? Move your body and make a withdrawal of cortisol (that thing that makes you feel crappy) and make a deposit of serotonin (that thing that makes you feel great). Our lifestyle, situations, and circumstances can be making deposits of cortisol into our body over and over and over. If we aren't balancing those deposits of cortisol with making deposits of serotonin, our bank account can be very low or overdrawn. When it is overdrawn, your body and your mind will start suffering. Put another way: if you don't make time for your mental wellness, you will be forced to make time for your illness.

When your mental health suffers, so does the rest of your body. While a panic attack can mimic signs of a heart attack, mental illness can also show up in serious physical health complications such as heart disease, high blood pressure, weakened immune systems, autoimmune diseases, asthma, obesity, and stomach problems. Perhaps improving your mental wellness will alleviate some other health concerns you are battling. Didn't think they were connected? Know now, they are all connected.

I have compiled a list of exercises that are great for anyone looking to improve their mental wellness:

1. **Any exercise**—Any at all is better than none. Recommendations here in Canada say adults between the ages of eighteen and seventy-nine should

get at least 150 minutes of moderate to vigorous exercise per week, but only 49% of that age group is achieving that target.[23] My own personal rule of thumb is thirty minutes a day. If I am having a bad mental health day, I increase it to forty-five minutes or an hour. I like to write down a daily total of how many minutes I get each day and total it at the end of the week. This is a really easy way to make sure you are getting enough. Other ways to track this is using a device like a Fitbit or Apple watch that can track your movement. It is important to note that older generations should also be striving for this kind of activity if able to do so. Activity levels should remain the same throughout our lifetime, as long as our bodies are able to tolerate it.

2. **Get outside**—Any time you are able to incorporate nature into your exercise, it will benefit your mental wellness. Research is growing in this field that is being called ecotherapy. Ecotherapy (being in nature) helps to reduce stress, anxiety, and depression. In a 2015 study, Harvard researchers compared the brain activity of healthy people after they walked for ninety minutes in either a natural setting or an urban one. They found that those who did a nature walk had lower activity in the prefrontal cortex, a brain region that is to blame for repetitive thoughts and negative emotions.[24] Natural sunlight can reset your circadian rhythm (your ability to sleep well) and also provides much-needed vitamin D. Deficiencies in vitamin D can contribute to mental illness and I will have more on that later because it is so important especially in Canada where we have limited daylight. Exercises you can do outside include swimming, walking, running, biking, kayaking, hiking, gardening, golfing, and many more. Find a reason to get outside. Better yet, I'll give one: your mental health!

3. **Yoga**—Yoga is next because of the quietness it teaches, the breathing techniques help to calm our bodies and minds, and the stretching. Yoga, while not a high-intensity workout, is a daily practice for me in addition to getting my thirty minutes a day. Yoga can help improve concentration by helping you move from the sympathetic nervous system to the parasympathetic nervous system, which means taking you from the fight-or-flight response to rest and digest. As soon as you start breathing deeply, you slow

down (out of fight or flight) and calm your nervous system, also lowering blood pressure. Yoga is a great way to stretch your muscles, especially if they are tense from worrying. It can also decrease inflammation and, as a result, reduce anxiety and depression.

4. **Dancing**—Dancing takes the number four spot because it takes your thoughts off anything else and focuses on how to move your body in a way that matches the music. And if you can dance to music that strikes a happy emotional response in your brain, you will get double the deposit in your serotonin bank account. Add to that, dance with a partner and you'll also get bonus points for connection and physical touch. Your serotonin bank account will be overflowing! So, kick up your heels. This feels like the right time to play a song.

CUE UP HAWG WYLDE'S "KICK OFF YOUR BOOTS"

Hawg Wylde is such a little-known Canadian band from my past but it brings back so many happy memories of dancing with my peeps back in the day. If you can find it (try YouTube), pretend you are from a small town (or maybe you are), surrounded by cowboys and cowgirls two-stepping to this nineties anthem in a sand-covered arena or patch of grass. The song ends with a really fast polka. I dare you to find a partner and try it. Honestly, this is some good medicine right here and I am writing you the prescription!

5. **What you do matters**—Don't exacerbate your condition. Some days you are going to feel like you are forcing yourself to move your body. I get that. And on those rough days when you are feeling mentally injured or mentally ill, it will absolutely feel like you are dragging your feet to get moving, and you will do it anyways (because now you know why it is important). But on a good mental health day, I want you to enjoy the activity you are doing. Find those things that fire you up. Find something that you look forward to doing. Maybe you enjoy going for a walk with your spouse, maybe you enjoy playing sports with your friends, maybe you really like playing Frisbee with your kids, and maybe you enjoy running alone with nobody around you but the sounds of nature or the music in your headphones.

Whatever it is that you enjoy doing, do that first. If you try a workout video and you absolutely hate it, don't do it again. Try something else. Some people enjoy the structure of a program like beach-body workouts because it lays out a plan for them and is regimented and predictable. Others want the freedom to pick what workout they want to do each day. Both work fine, as long as you have a plan in place and make it a habit into your daily activities. Mental wellness relies on habits and consistency.

What if you are unable to exercise? Maybe you are injured or elderly and can't move, then do whatever you can. If you can't move your legs, move your arms. If you can't move your arms, move your legs. If you can't move at all, the other mental health strategies I suggest should replace exercise (things like finding connection, good nutrition, and mindfulness to name a few).

Your ability to manage your mental wellness in terms of managing your thoughts and emotions starts with maintaining brain health, and the best way to do that is to move your body.

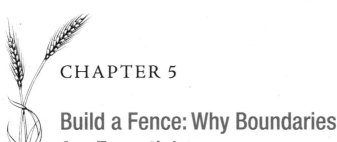

CHAPTER 5

Build a Fence: Why Boundaries Are Essential

If you own livestock, you know there is one rule that always holds true: the animals will always get out on a day when you have something planned. It is inevitable that if you have a wedding or graduation to attend, you will surely be taking off your high heels to go chase cows before attending the event, arriving late of course, and likely a bit sweaty from your obligations at home. Fences are important infrastructure on a farm or ranch just as boundaries are crucial for our mental health.

When we were first married, my husband James and I used to own cows. The fences on our pastures were often old, some of the strands of barbed wire had fallen down, and the posts had a lean to them. When the fences were new, they did a fantastic job at keeping the cows in and the predators out. However, over time, those fences degraded, and the structural integrity was no longer there. Slowly, predators started creeping in, and once in a while (usually on a day that we had something planned), the cows would get out. Fences are built for livestock for a very important reason, but without maintenance, those fences don't serve the purpose they were built for. The same can be said for the boundaries we have in our lives. We first need to know where to put them, but we also must know when to adjust them and maintain them when something is pushing on our fence. Triggers in our lives (things that cause us to have a strong emotional response) can threaten our mental health just as predators can threaten our livestock.

What are your triggers? You know the kind of things that makes you get tight muscles and hot in the cheeks, and your heart starts beating faster than you thought possible? That emotional response is stress on your body and mind. Some triggers are easy to identify: you are stuck in traffic, your bank account is overdrawn, you have a sick child on a day you planned an important meeting, or the Canada Revenue Agency (or IRS if you are American) call to do an audit.

Aren't those phone calls always the best? Ugh. Those are triggers you may not be able to control, but what about the ones we can prevent from happening? Some triggers may be affecting your mental health without you even realizing it. That's because you may have had them around for so long, maybe even for decades, that they have become normal to you. That doesn't mean they aren't causing strain on your mental health, but it does mean it might be harder for you to recognize them.

It has taken me years to recognize one of my biggest triggers for my mental health is feeling judged. It actually doesn't even have to be that someone is judging me. In fact, it can simply be my perception that someone is judging me. Making up stories in your head that differ from reality is a classic symptom of anxiety. And let me tell you, I could win an award at that. Besides feeling overwhelmed, this is the second biggest trigger for me. As a result, the most valuable relationships in my life are people whom I perceive (perception is the key here) as non-judgemental people (whether they are judging or not isn't really the point). It seems to be my perception that ultimately matters. I've had to first distinguish who truly is and isn't a threat to my mental health (and gosh, sometimes that is the hardest part if you are an overthinker.) Some of my best supports are in my family (my own kids are the best for this and will love me no matter what I do), but others are friends who I feel comfortable being vulnerable with. These are the kind of friends you can call up on a bad day and just have a cry about something or when you get off the phone with them, you feel so much better. They let you feel, they listen, and in return, you don't feel judged. However, when faced with a person who is constantly criticizing or judging something I am doing, that fence gets built pretty darn fast. I've also realized that people will always judge you if you are living bravely and authentically. I've learned that I have to be OK with my own decisions, regardless of what others think. This can be a hard one if you live with anxiety, but it has been a very important discovery. I am living my life for myself, not because of what other people think of me. Here is a great life hack: some people will mistreat you but it is your duty to get out of harm's way and do right by your own mental health.

That being said, if you have a relationship where you can give and receive without judgement, it is some of the best medicine so seek those out. And I'll talk more on this in chapter 10 because the importance of connection merits its own chapter. Without having someone that you can give and receive with judgement, it can be very isolating to deal with mental health issues alone. You can be in a relationship with someone and still feel very isolated. You can be surrounded by a support system, but if you don't feel genuinely supported, you can still feel isolated.

My husband never really understood my anxiety when I was living it at the beginning. To be honest, he can't totally understand it now although he has gotten a lot of education from me along the way. That doesn't mean he isn't a good support. If I say I didn't sleep well, he might help with the kids and let me go have a nap. If I say, "My chest is tight and my heart is racing," he'll usually offer a foot rub. When I need support, all I need my husband to say is, "What can I do to help you right now?" To be honest, there are a lot of times when I can't fully understand my own anxiety, so I can't really expect him to understand it either. I can go weeks feeling amazing and then all of a sudden feel overloaded with stress and anxiety. We all have times when we feel good and times when we are struggling. I'm still understanding all of my triggers, but that doesn't mean I can totally avoid them either. I'm just learning to recognize them and deal with them the best way I can to honour my mental health. So how can you do the same?

When we realize a certain trigger causes a strong emotional reaction, we can try and take a step back and say to ourselves, "How can I react to this feeling in a way that serves me?" Perhaps flying off the handle at someone who triggers us isn't always the best choice for our own mental health. Perhaps removing yourself from certain situations you know might trigger those reactions is also helpful. Perhaps a constant beeping phone sets you off: turn off the notifications for a while. Perhaps dealing with finances bothers you: set aside a specific time to look at them and then put them away. We can't escape all of our triggers but we can compartmentalize them, schedule some of them, and avoid others intentionally to prioritize our own mental health.

These things are called boundaries. Just like the fences on the farm protect our livestock, boundaries protect our mental health. If having a conversation with your brother-in-law about politics is going to set you off, perhaps you avoid those topics. If you have someone in your life who is always criticizing the way you do things, perhaps you stop them the minute they start to do it, and tell them you didn't ask for advice. Perhaps you avoid them if they don't stop. It is absolutely essential to put up a boundary with people, places, or things if you know that it will injure your mental health. No apology is required for doing so, and there is no guilt allowed when it comes to making boundaries for your mental health. I don't care if it is your sister, your cousin, or your best friend's husband.

Here is another fence analogy for the city folk in the crowd. Boundaries, when put in the right place, are like putting up a fence to keep out your neighbour's dog who keeps shitting on your lawn. The dog doesn't know any different, it just needs to take a shit. But when a fence is in place, the dog knows it can't doody on your green patch of backyard bliss anymore. The dog isn't really affected by the change because it still relieves itself anyways. The same can be said for setting boundaries with people, places or things. People may or may not notice, but they likely won't be affected by your additional space. You will, however, see a benefit to nurturing your mental health and avoiding those unhealthy triggers. Boundaries can look different for everyone. It can mean putting work away at 5:00 p.m. (this isn't always possible on the farm and maybe looks more like 7:00 p.m. or 8:00 p.m. or later in busy seasons), it can mean shutting your TV off a couple hours before bed and prioritizing sleep, it can mean saying no to another task you've been asked to take on when you are already overloaded, and it can even mean not going out on the town if you know that staying home is what you really need.

Farmers work where they live and live where they work. The mental escape from work does not exist as it does for people who go to a place of work at a physical location away from where they live. This lack of separation between work and home life can be difficult. To have a home that feels like a refuge, boundaries are acutely important. My husband and I have a boundary that we created a few years ago. When we are in the house for the evening, and the work is done for the day, we don't talk finances or any farming business after 10:00 p.m. If someone brings something up, we say, "Nope, it is after ten." We resume the conversation the next day. This boundary prioritizes a time in the evening for our relationship and for a quiet, calm brain before we go to bed, clearing our mind before we lie down for the night. Here are some other tips for establishing boundaries in conversation from The Do More Agriculture Foundation:

1. What you said wasn't funny to me. It was hurtful.

2. I need help/support/assistance. Can I please have help with _____.

3. I am speaking; please stop cutting me off.

4. Right now is not a good time for me to chat. Let's revisit this at a different time.

5. I have had a stressful day at the farm (or work); let's try this when I am refreshed.

6. I realized that you are going through something difficult. I don't feel equipped at the moment to help with this. Can I help you find the support you need?

7. It's not my place to discuss someone else's life.

8. I'm not ready to talk more about what I am going through. I need time to process.[25]

When looking for advice on being depressed, I've found that many people offer up connection as a solution. While I agree genuine connection is one of the most helpful tools, surrounding yourself with people isn't always the answer. You can surround yourself with people and still feel isolated. You can also sabotage yourself and have shallow conversations with people and that can also make you feel isolated if you yearn for deep, meaningful conversations. If you aren't being real about what you're feeling, and really trusting in the relationship, you might as well stay in bed under a blanket. One hundred people in a room won't matter if you can't have a meaningful conversation with one of them. If you are an introvert and work out things in quiet, then you can do that too—under a blanket recommended! If you are seeking connections, just be sure to build a fence when you need one.

There are so many other triggers for my anxiety, things like not enough exercise, not enough sleep, skipping meals or bad nutrition, a lack of time outside, or consuming alcohol. I make sure to limit how much alcohol I consume, or completely avoid it if I'm feeling a bit off with the awareness that it will make it much worse. There is evidence about the negative effects of what alcohol can do to our brains as we age. A study released in Scientific Reports in January 2020 reports that after studying the brains of over 11,500 deceased people, they found that drinking accelerated the age-related damage that degrades memory and intelligence. They concluded that just one gram of alcohol consumed per day ages the brain by roughly a week. [26]

When I avoid my triggers, I usually feel like my anxiety is manageable, but if one or two things trigger my anxiety, it can make everything seem out of control.

Knowing triggers can be one of the most helpful tools for prevention and maintenance. Do you ever sit around a campfire and there is always that one person that just disappears earlier than everyone else, sometimes mid-conversation? That's me. I'm that person. If I know that I need sleep to function the next day, I don't care if you want to stay awake all night long, but I'm going to hit the hay when I know it is time. If I've had enough socialization and just need alone time, I'm going to take it with no apologies required. That's my boundary. That's my fence.

You might relate with my next trigger: the desire for perfection. I don't think I am alone in this one and so I think it is important to share this with you. Anyone who struggles with high-functioning anxiety will know that you can be having a bad mental health day where you feel absolutely awful, but you will still drop off muffins at the school for the breakfast program, coach hockey, balance your bankbook, scrub toilets, and do every piece of laundry in the house, all while feeling like you were hit by a truck. If you are really good at being a perfectionist, you might even have your hair and makeup done and smile at everyone you encounter.

Being a perfectionist is a tricky trigger to pinpoint, or at least it was for me. I am very goal-driven and hard-working and have always been rewarded for doing my best. Society always rewards perfectionists. This is a great thing mostly for other people. Because if you are a go-getter, you know how to get shit done. People love having me on committees around the community because they know I will take the burden of the work and run with it. This can also lead to being taken advantage of by an employer, your family members, or friends. Being a perfectionist means that sometimes I have to finish a job at all costs, even if it means not listening to my body telling me to stop and take a break. It can also mean not starting a job or putting it off because of fear that I won't be able to do it perfectly. It means I can spend hours on something that doesn't actually matter, like the title of this book, the size of the font, or the way it is laid out, instead of focusing on the content. It can also put people off when they feel they can't live up to your ridiculous standards. I realize that not everybody wants to live with the kind of expectations I put on myself and I honestly don't blame them! I don't want to either!

Expectations can suck, especially our own! I grow a huge garden because I truly love gardening. My connection to the land is engrained in me, and I'm happiest when my hands are in the dirt. You know you are a farmer when you find sheer bliss in growing things. The calm and quiet of the garden, intertwined with the vines of produce, can be some of the best pleasure for me. But sometimes, in the middle of pickling season, I have to say to myself, "Put the canner away! That's enough." (My husband is pretty good at telling me to do the same, as much as he loves pickles.) Our society has been taught over decades that our worth is tied to how much we get done in a day. But it isn't. We aren't the sum of our tasks. We need to meet certain needs to live and to look after our family, and we still need to go to work and bring home a paycheque and maybe we still have to coach the hockey team, but maybe our schedules need to be more intentional about what we are doing and why we are doing them.

Let me put it this way: trim the fat and keep the meat. When the cucumbers are overflowing in the garden, and I've made enough pickles for the year, there is no reason to overdo it—the chickens get fed cucumbers instead. To conquer this part of my anxiety, I have adopted a new rule lately: I will do my best, but not at the expense of my mental health. If I see my mental health suffering I try to stop and say to myself, "Is this good enough?" Perhaps being good enough is better than being perfect. Perhaps the floor only gets vacuumed once a week instead of daily. Perhaps the bathrooms get scrubbed every second weekend instead of every weekend. Perhaps I only can thirty quarts of dill pickles instead of fifty. Perfect is a pretty big word to live up to and most things in life aren't that. So why do I have to be? It would be great if we had someone to tell us we don't have to move mountains every day. I now recognize I need to be that person. I need to say, "STOP! You are feeling overwhelmed." If you notice that you have these tendencies to do it all and be everything for everyone, try to tell yourself to stop and build that fence. Take a breath and evaluate where you are at often. Perfectionism is a trigger that can be hard to recognize but a really important one to tackle in order to improve mental health.

Any kind of health issue can trigger anxiety too. I know pretty quickly when I am getting sick with a cold or a flu because my anxiety is bad. It is a tell-tale sign. If you are doing everything to manage your mental health and still feel like crap, go see your family doctor because something else might be going on. I can't stress this enough: trust your gut. If you don't feel well, find out why. Too much caffeine, too much salt, and certain medications can also trigger my anxiety. Getting to know all of these triggers has taken years of listening to my body. It isn't an easy thing to recognize. It is mostly learned through trial and error and a whole lot of self-awareness.

What's your triggers? Perhaps your trigger is a long to-do-list. Perhaps the fear of the unknown. Do parties or social events make you uncomfortable? Identifying your triggers can prevent you from having a bad day even when circumstances are out of your control. Then, when you are feeling crappy, you can ask yourself: Did I sleep enough? Did I drink too much alcohol? Did someone say something to me that set me off? Did I drink enough water today? Did I eat properly? Becoming self-aware is the most powerful tool in our anxiety toolbox. When we learn how to listen to our thoughts and feelings and how it affects our body, it can guide us in the right direction: feeling good.

What about this one? Have I spent too much time on my phone? That's a legitimate question these days. Netflix has a documentary called The Social Dilemma that touches on this. If you haven't watched it, I recommend taking the time to do it. Setting boundaries with the electronics in our lives can make such a meaningful and positive impact on our mental wellness. We know they are here to stay, so be intentional about how you use them. We have rules in our house like no phones during meal time, none before school for the kids, and none before they have done their morning routine and chores on weekends, and absolutely none for at least two hours before bed. That leaves a small window they are allowed to be on devices: while they ride the bus or for a few minutes after school or on weekends. As adults running a farm, we need our phones to do business most of the day, but I try to be very intentional about how I use it. The only notifications that are turned on are calls and texts. No other notification will make noise because everything else is deemed non-urgent and just adds to unnecessary screen time throughout my day (and distractions). Being intentional about how you use your devices and limiting screen time will benefit your mental health. Prioritize real life connections over Internet connections. Everyone—not just my kids—can benefit from that. However, I think there is an important role for devices, Internet connections, and social media. If used properly, it can serve as connections for people who are lacking those face-to-face connections, they can serve as an educational tool, and let's be honest, it is great for businesses that don't have store fronts. Be device smart. If you find it is a trigger for you, then you may need to change your habits around them—aka build a fence!

There are so many triggers. I have named a few to get you thinking what triggers you might have. When you identify your triggers, it is easier to either restrict or avoid those things (alcohol, phones, negative people, unhealthy foods) or work to get more of what you need for mental wellness (exercise, healthy food, good support people).

While I already emphasized the absolute importance of exercise for your mental health, over the next few chapters I am going to lay out some good, easy-to-live-by rules of what else you will need to feel your best. Things like nutrition, sleep, self-care, hormone health, connection, mindset, confidence, and compassion.

Identifying your triggers is a learning process. Over time, you will become acutely aware of when you feel good and when you don't. Maybe you already know what your triggers are and maybe it will take some time. Maybe you have a trigger you didn't even realize was one, because you have been conditioned over time to believe that it is normal. I hope the next time you want to binge on salty food and alcohol, and it makes you feel like crap, you might think twice before doing it again. Setting boundaries can be a hard thing to do, but if you think of it as putting up a fence to keep threats to your mental health outside your emotional space, it becomes clear that they are essential to protecting your mental wellness.

Author Doe Zantamata has written a book series called *Happiness in Your Life*. One of my favourite quotes speaks to the idea of setting boundaries. "If someone asks you to do more and you have a big reaction inside, it may be a sign that you're already doing too much. Even strong, independent, hard-working people have limits and deserve to rest. Doing your best is a wonderful thing, but doing all you possibly can for as long as you possibly can will eventually lead to burning out and feeling unappreciated by the people around you."[27]

Your mental wellness is sacred. Build a fence around it.

CUE UP "FENCEPOSTS" BY CODY JOHNSON

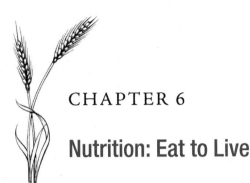

CHAPTER 6

Nutrition: Eat to Live

It's 2:00 a.m., I've been sitting in the seat of my combine for about sixteen hours, only leaving the cab briefly for bathroom breaks, and a quick meal over the tailgate of the truck.

After long workdays and little sleep during harvest on our farm, I seem to get hungrier by the second. For me, exhaustion goes hand in hand with hunger. Lack of sleep usually means I fall into bad eating habits. There is good reason for that. A 2012 study in the *Journal of Clinical Endocrinology and Metabolism* looked at the connections between sleep deprivation and cravings for high-calorie foods. It showed that the longer sleep deprivation lasts, the more cravings the participants experienced, usually leading them to consume unhealthier food and eat larger quantities.[28] The same thing occurred when I was sleep deprived with two small children. I was up three to four times at night breastfeeding, tending to a toddler with a bad dream or taking someone to the potty, and would get extra hungry. Hungrier than I've ever experienced in my life. Many nights I would have tackled an all-you-can-eat buffet at 3:00 a.m. if given the opportunity. What I didn't know then is that there is a reason for that hunger. Obviously, when you are breastfeeding, you need to increase your calories to produce milk, but being tired also played a huge roll in my desire to eat 24-7. It's the hunger hormone, ghrelin, which spikes when you are sleep deprived. I call it the *Gremlin* (like those little creatures in the 1984 movie) because once you feel it, it will haunt you and won't go away unless you get sleep.

When those same gremlins or hunger pains hit at harvest and I'm in the combine, my go-to snack in the cab of my John Deere used to be dark chocolate. All the dark chocolate! The combination of sugar and caffeine were a terrible combination. I would get a rush of energy and then feel grumpy, tired, and still hungry, not long after my sweet snack. I have realized that if I pack myself fruits and vegetables, along with some protein like nuts or seeds to snack on in the combine, I will feel fuller longer, alert, and not so grumpy—something the rest of the harvest crew is thankful for. Getting hangry (hungry and angry) is just one way that food can affect our mood, but everything we put in our body affects the way it works, especially our mind and ultimately our mental health.

Nutrition is something I am passionate about because I know nutrition is one currency we can use to buy ourselves better mental health (and overall health). In this chapter, I have tried to take what I have learned in the last five years and put it in just a few pages (which was super hard by the way and the toughest chapter to write), but the best tip I can recommend is to find replacements for the things you love to eat. This worked so great for me. There are so many ways to replace the not-so-healthy foods that you crave with a healthier option. I would much rather replace a once-in-a-while food than restrict it all together. That's because I love to cook and bake, and I love even more to eat good food. Baking is so good for my soul and I love sweets. I adore them! I want a sweet after every meal. No joke. If you have will power and don't need a sweet after every meal, then let's give you a shout-out right here and right now. Also, please teach me your ways! In the meantime, I'll be over here making black bean brownies and lentil chocolate chip cookie cake because if I trick my mind into thinking that I am indulging in something delicious, sweet, and savoury, then it is just as good as the real thing, but usually with less sugar and more protein.

This strategy of replacing foods with healthier options was trial and error for me. You have to be willing to try thirty recipes in order to take five or six that you would be willing to make again. I have made so many that were awful: there was the time I made zucchini tater tots that quickly got tossed to the dog, who also didn't want to eat them. However, the ones that were great are sticking around for life now, including zucchini pizza crust, pork and black bean chili, and a healthier version of pancakes with whole grains and flax that my kids love every Saturday morning. I want to challenge you to find what foods you love, that you know aren't serving your body with not-so-nutritious ingredients, and find a way to make them healthier. What's healthier? Lucky for you I have broken down some of the best information all in this chapter.

Anxiety loves sugar. So does depression. If you only do one thing to improve your mood, ditch the sugar. A 2017 study from London found that increased consumption of sugar can worsen mood disorders like anxiety and depression.[29]

While another study in 2019 links individuals without depression to a diet that consisted of more legumes, fruits, and vegetables.[30]

Science is backing up the idea that your digestive system guides your emotions. What you eat makes up the cells of your body and your brain and ultimately affects your mood from the moment it hits your lips. They say "You are what you eat," but it's funny, I don't remember eating a sexy beast this morning. OK, that joke was meant to make you laugh in a chapter that feels a lot like school but I'll put this in a very easy way to understand. What your mother said is true: everything in moderation—unless they are potato chips, then definitely cut that shit out. Nobody needs to eat potato chips. Better yet, continue supporting potato farmers and replace those chips with a baked potato!

Megan Shipp is a certified healthy eating coach with CanFitPro and is a guru when it comes to eating healthy. The early childhood educator and mom of three lost one hundred pounds over four years with a goal of being a healthier and happier mom. Her passion to help other women led her to get certified as a nutritionist herself. She now helps others, teaching clients to relearn how to eat in a way that fuels their bodies in order to feel their best. I couldn't think of anyone better to interview for this topic! Combining her advice and my own observations, I can tell you what foods will serve your body and, more importantly, your mind. Shipp says that having a goal of better mental health for changing your eating habits is a fantastic "why." Most people tell her they want to lose weight or get healthy, but she says, "The effects to your mental health are seen before the scale moves or your clothes fit better."[31] Nutrition should give you energy to get through your day without feeling groggy or having brain fog and should make you feel good from the inside out.

I know from experience, that if I eat crap, I will feel like crap. Before changing my eating habits, I thought I ate relatively healthy. After being coached on ways to improve my nutrition, I didn't realize how great I could feel, until I made some of these changes. My mood improved, I had more energy throughout the day, and I liked what I saw in the mirror too.

If you struggle with anxiety or depression, then basic nutrition and exercise are the two things you should be striving for every single day according to professional counsellor Erica Hildebrand who deals with many clients who struggle with mental illness. "In my opinion, exercise and healthy eating are among the top of my list of first things that I would suggest to someone struggling with anxiety," she says. So let's break it down in to a few easy guidelines.

1. **Eat regularly**—Do not skip meals. You brain will only work well if it is fueled with what it needs. If you aren't giving it what it needs, it simply cannot perform for you. When my son Lane started kindergarten, he would come home with his lunch still packed the way I packed it when he left for school in the morning: a sandwich, a piece of fruit, some veggies, and a granola bar. Sometimes he would eat a couple pieces of veggies, and sometimes nothing was touched. Do you know what kind of cranky human walks off the school bus when he hasn't eaten all day? A crying, emotionally distraught mess of a human. He would become a puddle on the floor when he got home from school until I could get some food into him. While a growing five-year-old needs to eat his lunch to grow and have energy, he also needs it for his mental health just as we do at any age. Your energy levels and mood will always be affected when you miss a meal. Make mealtimes a priority in your day.

2. **Water**—Dehydration affects cognitive functioning. Researchers at Tufts University did a study in 2009 that found dehydration can negatively affect mood. Participants in the study experienced fatigue, confusion, tension, and anger. Dehydration was also found to mimic the symptoms of anxiety: things like increased heart rate and dizziness. [32] So if you are feeling a bit off, go take a chug. Another study from the University of Connecticut found even mild dehydrations affects mood in healthy young women. [33] When I asked Shipp about other benefits to keeping your water jug close by, she says it is about more than just hydration: "Drinking water is also a simple chance to pause in your day and breathe in between the demands." Your entire body will thank you when you start drinking more water. Now put this book down and before you keep reading, go get out a water jug and fill it up. I'll wait. Got it? OK good, now take a big chug. Now attach said water jug to your belt, put it in your purse, backpack, and never leave home without it again. This will be your new best friend. This also means replacing whatever else you are drinking that does not serve your brain (coffee, alcohol, pop, energy drinks) and replacing it with water. If

you can't give up coffee, limit it to one cup a day. Coffee is a diuretic and has dehydrating effects, so for every cup of coffee you drink, two cups of water are needed to rehydrate your body. Drinking water is the best thing you can do for your body. Before you change your eating habits, increase your water intake first. (I am a believer in introducing one habit at a time.) Try drinking more water for a couple weeks, then stack on another habit. Sometimes trying to implement too much change at once can derail the best of intentions. Start with water and then work your way down this list.

I have a 2.5 L water bottle. I make sure I fill it up in the morning and make sure it is empty at night. It is huge and I carry it around everywhere. My friends and family make fun of me constantly about my big jug. It is a running joke that I drink lots and pee lots. But this one thing made such a huge difference in how I feel. It made me have less cravings for food I didn't need to be eating, it made my bowel movements more regular, which in turn, helped my stomach feel better, and it improved my hair, nails, and skin. Most importantly though, staying hydrated drastically improved my mood and decreased my symptoms of anxiety.

Your brain requires water to operate. How much? A good rule of thumb is drinking half your body weight in ounces each day. Drinking enough water will keep your brain cells active and balances chemical processes in the brain, helping to regulate stress and anxiety. If you don't have a large water jug, no problem! Grab a small one and at the beginning of the day put four elastics around it. Each time you fill it up during the day, take one elastic off. This way you will know how much you drank by the end of the day, and you can keep track of your refills.

3. **Vegetables**—The majority of your diet should be composed of vegetables. A great rule of thumb is to fill half your plate with vegetables. Your fridge should always be full of vegetables too. Ideally Shipp recommends aiming for three to six servings each day. When you go grocery shopping, your cart should look vibrant with green and other colourful vegetables. The greener, the better. Leafy greens like spinach, kale, and broccoli are rich in brain healthy nutrients like vitamin K, lutein, folate, and beta carotene. A study done at Harvard in 2018 linked certain foods to better brain power, suggesting that leafy greens may help slow cognitive decline. The study

found that even one serving a day will provide benefits.[34] But don't discount a good red pepper or a bag of carrots. When I wanted to eat healthier, I went to the store and bought any kind of vegetable that I couldn't pronounce, or I had never tried before. Then I found out how to eat it or cook with it and I tried new ones over and over again. Some of them were terrible (I can't stand eggplant!), but some of them I loved (spinach, spaghetti squash, red peppers). Try new vegetables and you might be surprised that you have been missing out. Have you tried arugula? How 'bout endive? Or kale? (I personally don't love kale as much as some other people do, but I have a friend who loves to make kale chips.) You might be surprised what intrigues your taste buds. For me, I have a spinach obsession. In fact, most mornings I have a spinach and red pepper omelet. At first, my kids and my husband would turn up their nose at it. However, everything I made, I would make them try, and eventually this became a staple for breakfast in our house. I never would have eaten this before my healthy eating discovery but now it is my absolute favourite thing to eat in the morning and it leaves me feeling amazing.

How can you get more vegetables in your life? Find a store with a great produce section, visit a farmer's market, or grow it yourself. If you have the space and the time to garden, it can be the most rewarding way to spend your time. It is also a very easy way to keep lots of vegetables close at hand. And double points for your mood when you grow your own vegetables because there is growing evidence that gardening can benefit our mental health. A report in the Mental Health Review Journal says gardening helps reduce stress and improve mood, naming the hobby as a great mental health intervention.[35]

4. **Make protein a priority**—There are two kinds here: plant protein and animal protein. You should be getting both. Why? Because proteins are the main building blocks of your body. They're used to make muscles, organs, tendons, and skin, as well as enzymes, hormones, neurotransmitters, and other important components in our bodies that help them to function, including our brain.

Plant protein consists of nuts, seeds, and legumes. Almonds are great for a snack. Grab a few for a mid-morning or mid-afternoon snack. I love to have a tablespoon of raw pumpkin seeds beside my omelet each morning. I put flax in everything. If I am making bread or pancakes, flax goes in. Also, if I am making any kind of healthy baking, flax gets thrown in. Flax is an oilseed grown here on the prairies (and many other places too) that packs a punch. It is high in omega-3 (the good fats), lignans (which has antioxidant qualities), and fibre. Cooking with legumes like lentils are also great and is a great way to support our Canadian farmers too! There are so many options when it comes to nuts, seeds, and legumes but avoid salted or roasted nuts. Make sure they are raw to get the most benefit. And if you are eating peanut butter or other nut butter, make sure there is no added sugar. Have you eaten quinoa? Another one of my favourites is quinoa cooked in chicken broth or coconut milk instead of water. It is a dream!

Animal protein gives you more bang for your buck because it is a higher quality protein than plant protein. Meat is the most nutrient-dense food we can eat because it provides all the essential amino acids that our body can't produce on its own. Animal protein can also include dairy, eggs, or lean protein like chicken, turkey, pork, and fish. I don't want to discount beef here. A lot of healthy eating recommendations say that beef doesn't belong. I'm here to tell you that is does. My sister-in-law raises cattle on our farm and our freezer is usually always full of beef so we eat lots of it. Nutritionists have spent years debating the benefits of eating red meat. So far, the results have been mixed. However, any red meat, including beef, is a nutrient-dense source of protein and includes vitamin B12 and iron. Portion size for animal protein should be about the same size as the palm of your hand. More consistent protein (making sure there is protein at all three meals) should get you to a target of about fifty to one hundred grams of protein a day minimum. Shipp recommends 0.7 to 1.0 gram of protein per pound of body weight, so eat the damn meat!

Protein sources of all kinds provide amino acids which can improve your mood. Shipp says protein is essential in producing that happy hormone serotonin. "Tryptophan, an amino acid that is found in high protein foods, gets converted to serotonin in your brain. Eating foods with high levels of tryptophan also have other amino acids and together they can get to your brain." So make sure you are getting enough protein to produce the serotonin that you need.

5. **Healthy Fats**—We need fat to absorb the nutrients in our food. That's why at least 30% of our daily diet needs to be comprised of fat or 0.4 grams per pound of body weight. But not all fats are equal. We need healthy fats. Things like omega-3, -6, and -9—also known as brain food. Omega-3, specifically, is fantastic for helping your brain function and is found in foods such as fish and flax. Recent studies have shown that people already taking anti-depressants, as well as fish oil supplements with omega-3 saw greater improvements.[36] Preliminary research suggests it may be related to their effects on serotonin - the happy hormone that stabilizes our mood. It may also be attributed to its anti-inflammatory effects.

Here is another plug for Canadian farmers. We grow a lot of canola on the prairies, and over the past forty years, canola has become one of the most important oilseed crops worldwide. Canola oil is good for brain health because it provides the correct levels of omega-6 and omega-3 fats with a ratio of two to one.

Omega-9 sources can include olive oil, almond oil, walnuts, animal fat (yes lard!), and avocados. It isn't as important as the omega-3 and -6 because our bodies can produce omega-9 on its own, but the benefits of all these fats is a reason to add them into your diet. Butter, in moderation, is also a great way to get your healthy fats and it is also great for your colon to trade in that margarine for butter, canola oil, olive oil, avocado oil, flax oil, and hemp oil.

It is also important to mention coconut oil because there has been a lot of discussion on whether or not it should be part of a healthy diet. Coconut oil can certainly be included as a healthy fat in moderation because of its anti-inflammatory properties. Coconut oil can also help you burn fat, reduce hunger, and increase memory and brain function. Research from the University of Oxford shows that it may aid in the treatment of Alzheimer's.[37] Coconut oil can boost ketone production in the body (a fatty acid), which can improve cognitive function. I love coconut oil for all these reasons, plus it tastes amazing! However, coconut oil is also comprised of 90% saturated fat. Too much saturated fat can raise our bad cholesterol; however, coconut oil is also found to raise our good cholesterol. So, while coconut oil should be part of your diet, it should be used in moderation.

Let's not forget about our dairy farmers as well. Full fat options should be the preferred choice according to Shipp. While dairy does have saturated fat, it also provides good cholesterol. Full fat dairy products are a rich source of nutrients. Many times, low-fat products are loaded with extra sugar and other filler ingredients, so go for that high fat Greek yogurt, sour cream, or cream cheese! Shipp says, "The full fat option will leave you feeling fuller longer." She adds, "Our bodies cannot recognize the chemicals in processed fats like margarine and therefore stores them as sugar in our body. The food world demonized fat years ago and led people to believe that fat makes you fat, when the real culprit turned out to be sugar or eating more than we need to function. Taking the fat out of foods makes you consume more than you would in the full fat version and adds more sugar to your diet, which leads to spikes in insulin, crashes, and weight gain."

Keep a variety of fats in your diet to ensure you absorb the nutrients your body requires.

6. **Fruits**—Some healthy eating experts will often say fruit is very high in sugar and must be limited. Listen here. If you are going to eat fruit over any other kind of crap, then eat the damn fruit! The rule in my house is if you need a snack, raid the fruit bowl before you go into the pantry. Many times, you will get more nutrients that way, albeit with a bit more sugar content. The nutrients you will get from fruit will almost always outweigh the natural sugar content. A study in the *Journal of Nutritional Biochemistry* suggests that vitamin C, a well-known antioxidant, may play an important role in combating mood disorders.[38] So, load up on citrus fruit or berries whenever you can!

7. **Carbs** are brain fuel. Carbs are our friends. It has become a trend to cut out carbs in our diets, when in fact they should make up around 50% of our daily calories. Those carbs can come in a variety of forms, including something we grow a lot of: wheat. Unless you are gluten intolerant or celiac, which means you can't tolerate eating a protein found in wheat, barley, and rye, you should be eating wheat or other whole grains as part of your daily carbs as well as fruits and vegetables. Gluten has taken on a bad name lately. Gluten can cause bloating, digestive issues, skin rashes, and joint pain but only in a small percentage of the population (6 to 7%)

according to a study from the University of Maryland.[39] Lately, gluten has been marketed as something to stay away from, but humans have consumed grains for hundreds of years providing people with fibre, nutrients, and protein. Approximately 15% of the world's calorie intake comes from wheat.[40] We grow (and eat) a lot of wheat on our farm, but eating any kind of whole grains are great, as long as they are not overly processed. As soon as grains are processed or stripped down, a lot of the good stuff like fibre gets taken out. I don't mean get your grains in the form of a donut; I mean getting it in things like whole grain bread or whole grain pasta. One to two servings a day is all you need of whole grains. Too much can make you feel sluggish. That's because carbohydrates elevate your blood sugar, causing your body to have short bursts of energy followed by a crash or feelings of exhaustion. If you are eating bread, noodles, or crackers, make sure that they have whole grains.

Carbs don't just come from grains though. Foods like a baked potato, banana, beets, or blueberries will fill your carb requirement as well. *Do not eliminate carbohydrates.* They play an important role for our mental health. Health Canada recommends between 210 and 290 grams of carbohydrates a day. However, the National Academy of Sciences in the US recommends at least 130 grams, which is the minimum requirement for our brain to function. Carbohydrates help release that happy hormone, serotonin, which is why you might feel so happy when you eat that slice of bread! It really doesn't take much to meet your daily carb requirement. For example, a bowl of oatmeal (half a cup) contains twenty-seven grams of carbs. A baked potato has sixty-three grams of carbs. Eat your carbs and your brain will thank you.

8. **Whole foods**—From whole grains to whole food. If this all sounds like too many rules, then here is a good easy rule to remember: eat foods that are not processed. If it is in its original state, then it is probably good for you. Vegetables, fruits, seeds, and nuts are all good foods. If something is heavily processed, then it likely won't fuel your body the way it should. Sure, potato chips and French fries are potatoes, but being deep fried in oil and smothered in salt are reducing the true benefits it could offer. If you are eating meat, make sure it is a lean cut, not cured, salted, or heavily processed.

9. **Beneficial bacteria**—A healthy gut can mean you feel happier. A 2016 study in the *Journal of Psychiatric Research* found that if you transfer gut bacteria from a clinically depressed person into a rat, the rat becomes depressed.[41] What does that say about what is lurching in our bodies? The brain-gut connection is because of the gut's production of hormones and neurotransmitters like dopamine and serotonin. We need beneficial bacteria in our bodies to produce those things. Probiotic foods such as kombucha, sauerkraut, and other fermented foods can provide the kind of bacteria your stomach needs, and it may, in fact, help alter your mood. It can also help with bowel movements and eliminate stomach aches and pains by improving digestion. All of the tips I have offered will mean nothing if you don't have good digestion. It is the core component that must work with good nutrition in order to help you feel good. If you often have stomach aches, diarrhea, or constipation, locate a specialist that can help evaluate what foods you should or shouldn't be eating, because gut health is the basis for your entire body's health and especially your brain health.

Nutrient-dense foods are going to nourish your body and your mind. This does not mean you are going to lose weight. Please don't be confused. The only way to lose weight is to follow the law of thermodynamics. Fitness guru Jillian Michaels does a great job of explaining the law of thermodynamics. She has many videos on YouTube you can access if you want to learn more about this, I recommend one called "Will the CICO Diet help you lose weight?" Michaels explains that fat on our body is simply stored energy. Calories are a unit of energy. So if you eat more energy (calories) than you burn in a day, you will store that energy as fat. If losing weight is one of your goals, that simply means eating less and moving more. But she also explains that the quality of your food pertains to your health.[42] When eating to improve your mental health, quality of your food is the absolute most important thing. Remember what goes in your mouth ultimately makes up your brain cells, so feed your brain only the good stuff.

The guidance I have laid out here is to get you eating quality foods that will help with heart health, brain health, and overall wellness, if paired with exercise. If losing weight is your end game, then you might need to find resources on portion sizes. You may also want to figure out how many calories you burn in a day, and how many you are eating in a day. Creating a deficit is the only way to lose weight, if that is your end game. There are many programs that help to do that. (MyFitnessPal app was a good one for me.) But for the purpose of this book, please understand that these nutrition rules, paired with exercise, are meant solely for your mental wellness, not weight loss.

> Be aware that some mental illnesses like depression or anxiety can be directly related to a food allergy or intolerance. While these tips will guide you to eat for mental health, please be aware that if you don't feel right when eating a certain food, always be aware of that and take steps to avoid it or consult a professional before you take any further steps.

Changing the way I eat has been a difficult transition for me. It takes a lot of time to plan healthy meals and do meal prep with fresh whole foods. Processed foods are faster, no doubt, but the reward in preparing nourishing meals has been extremely rewarding and beneficial to my mental health, giving me energy, making me think clearer, and sleep better. If there is one takeaway from all of the nutrition talk let it be this: sugar will always be the biggest culprit when it comes to affecting your mood. Dr. Wendy Davis is a small town naturopathic doctor with a wealth of knowledge on all things health, and is another expert I asked to weigh in. She says cutting out sugar can make the biggest difference because, "sugar directly effects mood in the same way cortisol effects our brain."[43] Dr. Davis explains how we have evolved from a time when we had to run away from physical danger: "Increased cortisol happened when we were running away from lions and tigers and so it would fuel the muscles and the brain as a survival mechanism." She explains that stressors (psychological threats) can do the same thing to our body, releasing cortisol. Interestingly, eating sugar can have the same effect too: "Blood sugars go up but then they crash," she says. It is that crash that Dr. Davis says can influence our mood. Eliminating sugar can be uber helpful to regulate our blood sugar levels and, in turn, our mood.

A healthy, well-balanced diet cannot compete with high levels of stress or lack of sleep. Please hear me when I tell you that you cannot exercise your way to good mental health if you aren't eating properly. Too much exercise and poor nutrition can also make you feel rotten to the core. Taking supplements or drinking shakes should not replace good nutrition. They should only be used to complement a good diet. It is also important that nutrition is paired with good sleep habits and exercise to achieve mental wellness. Nutrition must come first, and supplementation can be added later if your body is not absorbing the micro-nutrients (vitamins and minerals) it needs from the food you are eating. Asking a naturopath or nutritionist to help you identify what micronutrients your body requires can be a good way to find out what you need, if any at all. Guessing at what vitamins and minerals you need might affect your health worse if you aren't taking the proper things or the proper dose.

When looking at macronutrients in your diet (carbohydrates, proteins, and fats), you should aim for a ratio of 50% carbohydrates, 30% fats, and 20% proteins. I recommend these percentages only because I know this works for me. I feel my best mentally and physically when I follow these guidelines. Adjustments to these might be needed, depending on your activity level and body needs. And of course, a professional opinion or appointment with a nutritionist or physician is always a good idea.

As with everything I recommend for mental wellness, make sure you are giving yourself grace. Don't obsess over what you are eating. Learning these guidelines take time. I am four and a half years into changing my eating habits, and I still find it easy to fall back into old habits, but the more I practice healthy eating, the easier it gets. Do I still go to Pizza Hut occasionally and enjoy a greasy pepperoni pizza? Absolutely. Do I eat a pancake and a couple slices of bacon on a Saturday morning with my family because it is my kid's favourite thing to eat? Absolutely. But the rest of the week I am being consistent about making sure I am getting what my body needs for my brain and my body to function well. My mental health requires nutrition, and so does yours.

CUE UP "CHICKEN FRIED" BY THE ZAC BROWN BAND

This song is just for fun. If you like your chicken fried, give yourself some grace and have some fried chicken once in a while. Don't ever associate feeling guilt or attempt to punish yourself for eating something you know isn't the best choice. Do your best and appreciate that as long as you are following these rules eighty percent of the time, you will see a benefit in your mental health, your energy, and your mood.

A Special Note about Supplements
Prescription Medication versus Adaptogens

No matter how clean your diet, you might still have to take prescribed medications to help you feel healthy and balanced. Again, this is something to consult and keep open communication with your physician about. And remember, there is no shame in needing these. The most widely used anti-depressants prescribed for depression and anxiety are selective serotonin reuptake inhibitors (SSRIs). SSRIs slow the reabsorption of the neurotransmitter serotonin to the brain. Drugs like Prozac, Zoloft, Paxil, Celexa, and Lexapro to name a few. Other prescription drugs include benzodiazepines—Xanax, Valium, and Ativan—that are tranquilizers and are used for anxiety. Most doctors will recommend prescription drugs in addition to therapy for best results. However, because of possible side effects and the potential for withdrawal when getting off these drugs, some people are hesitant to take prescription drugs. These drugs can play an important role if your anxiety and depression is at a critical stage, and getting treatment, in any form, is essential when mental illness becomes a barrier to carrying out daily tasks.

Please know that your doctor can help you find the right prescription drug for your symptoms and always be sure to get medical help if you are in a bad place mentally.

I have taken prescription drugs throughout my journey when necessary but have found other options as well. If prescription medication is something you are hesitant to take, another option is using adaptogens, supplements offered through holistic medicine. Naturopath Dr. Wendy Davis says they give people another option when dealing with mental health issues for those who are reluctant to take prescription drugs. "Adaptogens are where it's at. They are great for stress, energy and moods."

A relatively new nutrition supplementation for mental health, adaptogens are herbs that aid our bodies in reacting to or recovering from physical or mental stress. They do just as their name says by helping our bodies to adapt. Research conducted in Sweden in 2010 is gaining traction in the health world. Researchers believe that adaptogens work like a mini stress vaccine: helping to combat fatigue, enhance mental performance, and increase resistance to stress, in turn, easing anxiety.[44]

Just as prescription drugs treat anxiety or depression by balancing neurotransmitters in our brain, certain supplements may do the same.

5-HTP, tyrosine, taurine, and L-theanine are just a few that naturopathic doctors can recommend.

I take a daily supplement of magnesium with L-taurine and have seen positive effects on my sleep, mood, and bowel movements. (If you are a high-stress person, you may struggle with achieving these on a daily basis as well.) I also take vitamins B6 and B12 daily. Upon a live blood analysis, I discovered that I was deficient in B12 and since supplementation, I have found I have a lot more energy throughout the day. A new study revealed that magnesium paired with vitamin B6 can have more stress reduction in patients with low magnesium,[45] yet it is estimated that approximately 50% of Americans consume less than the estimated average requirement for magnesium, a mineral that is so crucial to our health.[46] Magnesium supports thyroid function, regulates cortisol, and helps with sleep, energy production, immune function, and hormone balance. It can even improve blood sugar and insulin sensitivity. Physical or mental stress can deplete magnesium from the body and is perhaps why it produces measurable benefits to people who take it. When paired with B6, magnesium may also help with anxious feelings and overall quality of life. These two supplements have become a daily staple in my life.

I also take a daily dose of curcumin, derived from turmeric and paired with black pepper extract for absorption. Some of the potential benefits include reducing inflammation, increasing circulation, as well as reducing depression and boosting brain function. The supplements I take benefit me, however, they may not work the same for everyone. That's why supplements and adaptogens need to be customized to your specific needs. Everyone has different needs, and supplements or adaptogens should be identified for specific patients, prescribed to meet individual needs, and should always be done with the help of a medical professional.

Curcumin works well for me because at a young age I was diagnosed with Raynaud's syndrome, which is a condition that decreases blood flow to extremities like fingers and toes. I am always susceptible to frost bite regardless of what mitts or boots I wear in the winter. Bad circulation, I've discovered, particularly in the brain, can be linked to depression and anxiety. Brain circulation is improved with exercise, which is perhaps why I find exercise one of the best cures for my anxiety and why curcumin is another helpful tool in my mental health toolbox. Finding the supplements that countered my body's shortfalls has been extremely helpful. If you have no problems with circulation or your lymphatic system as I do, you may not find benefits from this one like I have; however, naturopathic medicine individualized to the patient can identify which supplements may be able to complement your existing mental health routines. Another great one I rely on is an adaptogen blend called "Cortisol Calm." It is a great one to take when I'm in a period of high stress that I cannot control. It helps me calm down, get a better sleep, and overall feel better equipped to handle the tough stuff.

If you are interested in finding out more about adaptogens, talk to a naturopath doctor who can help you find out which ones are best for you and can also instruct you on a proper dosage. You can take adaptogens as herbal supplements in capsule form, or you can add them to smoothies, teas, or soups. They are a good tool to aid your body's brain chemistry but should never be used as a replacement to healthy foods that will nourish your body. Supplements should help nutrition but never replace it.

Adding nutritious meals into a busy schedule has been one of the toughest tasks to conquer. For example, as I write this, we are finishing up putting fall fertilizer down on our farm. I have been delivering meals for a couple weeks now, while my husband and nephew run our anhydrous units. That means I am single parenting at home while keeping up with the demands of school activities, lunches, laundry, and farm accounting. I recognize that I am growing increasingly tired of the schedule, and so last night before I crawled into bed, I made sure to find a crock pot recipe I could use this morning, because while I run my daughter to volleyball practice and my son to town for a birthday present he'll need for a birthday party tomorrow, supper needs to be cooking and ready when I get home. I know I could pick up a bucket of fried chicken in town for supper (and sometimes I do), but I also know that if I pre-plan a healthier option and get it started before we need to eat, I can tackle the rest of my day and know that our supper will be ready for delivery to the field when I return. My whole family will eat a healthier meal which will make all of us less cranky, feel full, and satisfied at the end of a busy day. It takes being a little more intentional, but the rewards are worth it when I have enough energy to deliver supper to the field, do cleanup, get the kids ready for bed, and finish my chores for the day instead of feeling like collapsing on the couch mid-way through the day.

Food is fuel. Plain and simple. Brain food is every food you put in your mouth, so make sure you feed it the best you can! Author of *The Hippocrates Diet and Health Program: A Natural Diet and Health Program for Weight Control, Disease Prevention, and Life Extension*, Ann Wigmore, said it best, "The food you eat can be either the safest and most powerful form of medicine or the slowest form of poison."[47]

I know this chapter had a lot of technical information but stay with me. Let's keep rolling, shall we?

CUE "ROLLIN'" BY BIG & RICH

Because who doesn't enjoy a song that has Cowboy Troy rapping about potato salad?

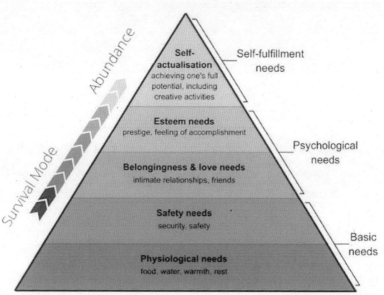

Maslow's Hierarchy of Needs

Self-fulfillment needs

Self-actualisation
achieving one's full potential, including creative activities

Esteem needs
prestige, feeling of accomplishment

Belongingness & love needs
intimate relationships, friends

Psychological needs

Safety needs
security, safety

Physiological needs
food, water, warmth, rest

Basic needs

Abundance

Survival Mode

Image courtesy of: @letstalk.mentalhealth

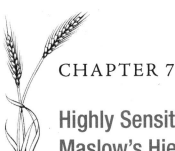

CHAPTER 7

Highly Sensitive People, Maslow's Hierarchy of Needs, and How It Can Help You Get to Sleep

The more tools you have on your journey to wellness, the better equipped you will be to reach your goal: feeling balanced, healthy, and sane. So where should you start? Maybe you have heard the term "survival mode." This comes from a psychologist named Abraham Maslow in a paper he wrote in 1943 called, "A Theory of Human Motivation."[48] We hear people say "survival mode" all the time, but do we really know what it means? Take a look at Maslow's hierarchy of needs, on the opposite page. It is a great visual to guide you when you are not sure where you are on your mental health journey.

Professional counsellor Erica Hildebrand has many clients that express being overwhelmed with anxiety and says, "Anxiety tends to have lots of layers. It's like pulling back the skin of the onion to get to what is really at the core of a person's anxiety disorder or mental health which may take differing levels of care." She says sleep, exercise, eating well, and limiting drugs and alcohol are all great places to start but adds counselling is necessary to help peel those layers back. "It's also evident that people who talk to a professional counsellor about what it is that brings them anxiety tend to feel fewer symptoms because what they may have kept hidden or never realized was the issue is now brought into the light, validated, and heard." While there are many tools to access on a journey to mental wellness, the best place to start is at the bottom of Maslow's hierarchy of needs—starting with your most basic needs.

When you are feeling overwhelmed, defeated, or unable to move forward, the best advice is to start at the bottom of this pyramid: our physiological needs like water and food (staying hydrated and nourished by healthy food). Going back to the basics and making sure you have those things covered is a great place to start. In fact, it is the only place you should start! Once you have covered these needs, then you can move up to the next level, making sure you are secure and safe (you have a place to live and are not worried for your safety). If you are living on the street and only worried about getting your next meal, you obviously are not concerned with your emotional needs as much as your physical required needs for survival, and you shouldn't be! Nor should you be worried about hanging out with friends or doing something creative if you are having trouble just getting out of bed and getting showered each day. While those things are all part of being mentally well and I would argue are the most rewarding when you get higher up the pyramid, I want you to understand that the basics *need* to be met first. That is why I am writing an entire chapter on sleep, something that might seem routine and obvious. But for anyone who is challenged by anxiety or depression, sleep can be anything but routine.

As a young mom, when I would wake up in the night when insomnia plagued me, just being awake fed my anxiety. I would wake up trembling, and even when able to calm myself down from a mid-night panic attack, I would still lie awake worrying about falling back asleep. With anxiety, I found that my desire to control everything, even my sleep, was the very root of the anxiety, a fear that I could not control it. Then I started wearing my Fitbit to bed and examining the chart of how little sleep I got each night. I would obsess over getting sleep, and in turn, feed my anxiety and ultimately get less of what I needed.

I knew that obsessing over sleep wasn't making it any better. So I surrendered and decided I would accept my sleep for whatever it was. I sold my Fitbit. I hated it for making my sleep worse. (I did buy another one a few years later and I absolutely love it for working out, but never wear it to bed.) I knew that nothing was ever permanent (this realization has been helpful for my anxiety as well—the only constant is change) and that if my sleep was going to be terrible for a while, I would accept that, but I also kept trying other things to see what made my nights better, and ultimately, my days too when I finally would get some shut eye. The less I worried about my lack of sleep, the better it got. That meant taking some advice and discarding others. There are so many personal development or motivational speakers that recommend getting up an hour earlier than you normally do and take time for yourself. I love a good motivational speaker but let me be clear about this kind of advice. It is great advice for people who are getting enough sleep, but if you aren't, take that tip and toss it. The 5:00 a.m. Club is not meant for everyone and definitely not meant for every stage of life, especially when you are tending to children throughout the night. It can also lead to burnout quickly. You absolutely should be making time for yourself in each day. However, you are not required to do it in the morning, or evening, or any particular time that will deprive you of sleep, one of your most basic needs. While taking time for yourself is crucial for your mental wellness, making sleep a priority should *always* come first.

My usual wake up time is between 6:30 and 6:45 a.m. in the winter. In the summer months, when we have earlier sunrises here in Manitoba, I love to get up with the sun. However, in general, I have tried to get up earlier as directed by other self-help gurus preaching success and doing it all and starting early each day. What I found was that my mental health does not benefit from super early mornings. It wasn't just me it was affecting either, but also the other people who live in this house alongside me. If I don't get around eight hours of sleep, my kids and my husband suffer in the evening when I am a grouch from about the supper hour right up to bedtime. Getting up earlier just wasn't good advice for me. It simply degraded the rest I needed and ultimately my mental health. Having said that, I do take an hour to myself during the day, but it does not mean getting up any earlier. Recognize what works for you. Some people thrive on five hours of sleep. I read a recent article that said Dolly Parton gets up at 3:00 a.m. to start her morning routine. Are you like Dolly? Or are you like me? Neither is wrong. That's because we all have a basal sleep requirement. Your basal sleep requirement is how much sleep you need for optimal performance, how much will get you through the day while functioning in a reasonable manner—that is, not being exhausted by suppertime.

I've recently learned that there is a group of people classified as highly sensitive people (HSP). When I learnt of this term, and read more about it, I immediately knew I was one of them. A great resource that I've found is a website called Highly Sensitive Refuge: A Community for Highly Sensitive People. According to the description on the page, being an HSP means, "Your nervous system is more sensitive to stimuli of any kind. That includes lights and sounds, but also things like subtle cues in body language or tone of voice." It goes on to say that highly sensitive people don't just notice more, their system processes it longer and more deeply. That means that almost any experience they have gets turned over in their mind again and again. As a result, HSPs are more prone to overstimulation and becoming overwhelmed."[49]

What does this mean when it comes to sleep? I've learned that my brain works in overtime to process this all and that my brain gets tired, often before my body does, and especially when there are lots of distractions or lots of things going on around me. It can increase my cortisol levels that can make my body feel like it is on high alert. I've learned that I get exhausted easily because of this, and that good quality sleep is the best medicine. Unfortunately, HSP find it more difficult to wind down and get sleep and stay asleep (also me), which requires a calm period before bed with little to no stimulation in order to catch those zzzz's.

If you thrive on five hours of sleep, you are free to get up at 4:00 a.m., assuming you have a bedtime of around 11:00 p.m. But if your basal sleep need is eight hours (like mine), you may need to hit the hay around 10:30 p.m. and wake around 6:30 a.m. Adjustments to that time depend on your needs, your work schedule, or your family's work or school schedule.

Let's be realistic though. While I strive for 8 hours every day, that isn't always achievable during certain seasons when you are a farmer. When it is seeding or harvest time on the farm and we are working long hours, I can get two to three hours a night. But when those days hit, I make sure that I pay off my sleep debt when the work is done. If it rains or if we are done our work and I am able, I will sleep for nine to ten hours for a few nights to make up for the loss that incurred during that time. Sneaking in a nap during the day to get another half hour also works. It doesn't matter how you catch up on your sleep debt. All that matters is that you do.

The same can be said for people who work shift work. If you are working shift work, you obviously can't be going to bed at the same time every day. So as long as you are meeting your body's basal sleep requirement and you are paying off your sleep debt when you can, those are the best things you can do for your mental health. While a regular sleep schedule is best for your body and mind, there are circumstances when we can't always get that. If you make up the difference where you can, then your physical and mental health will benefit because of it.

Signs that you aren't getting a quality sleep include:

1. Trouble falling asleep: if it takes you more than thirty minutes to fall asleep

2. Trouble staying asleep: waking up frequently

3. Waking up earlier than normal: waking up before you feel rested

4. Excessive fatigue: being tired throughout the day on a regular basis

5. Sleeping too much: this can be a sign that you aren't getting the REM sleep your brain requires. It may also mean you could have sleep apnea, which should be investigated by a doctor

Under-sleeping and over-sleeping disrupt our natural circadian rhythm, forcing our bodies to work harder. While not getting enough sleep can leave us feeling sluggish throughout the day, too much sleep can do the same thing. Keeping a regular bedtime and wake schedule, even on weekends, helps your body to know when it is time to sleep and time to wake.

Here's what's worked best for me:

1. **Make sure your room is dark**—A dark room signals your body to start producing melatonin, that great stuff in your body that makes you sleepy. Too much light, or light at the wrong time of day, will mess with that production. Lowering the lights before bedtime can help trigger that production.

2. **No screen time two hours before bed**—If you can't sleep, do not reach for your phone, or turn on the TV, as anything with a bright light will stimulate your brain and mess with your circadian rhythm.

3. **No caffeine or alcohol throughout the day**—I've read conflicting advice on when you should or shouldn't drink caffeine throughout the day and how much. But I can tell you, as someone who is super sensitive to caffeine, any amount will affect your sleep. Only you can decide how much you can tolerate. A good rule of thumb is this: caffeine has a half-life of five hours, which means that if you drink two cups of coffee at 9:00 a.m., the effects of that will last until 2:00 p.m. However, caffeine later in the day can really rob you of precious sleep. And if you are drinking a cup of coffee each morning and still finding that you aren't getting quality sleep at night, then get rid of that cup of coffee and see if it makes a difference. You might be cranky

for the first few weeks, but I will assure you that any amount of caffeine can steal precious sleep from you.

Alcohol and drugs can be the same. I think exercise is the most underused anxiety drug, while alcohol is the most accepted and overused anxiety drug in society. I used to drink wine every Monday night as I watched *ABC's The Bachelor or Bachelorette*. I convinced myself that it was part of my self-care routine (let me assure you it was not). I would relax for an hour of TV, but lose hours of sleep during the night because I indulged in some wine. Even one glass of wine will affect my sleep and to be quite honest, I just don't think it is worth it. Dr. James Rae is a general practitioner who works in rural Manitoba and works with many patients who struggle with alcohol addiction and mental health issues. I interviewed him on the topic and asked him how alcohol can play a role in worsening our mental state. He says a lot of people turn to alcohol for its sedating effects but it can degrade a patient's mental health as well as their quality of sleep. "Alcohol has a number of detrimental effects on mental health," he says. "One of the main ones being that it tells your brain cells not to talk to each other. It actually means that you need more signal to make any given brain cell fire in response to the chemical signals from other brain cells that are coming in. So what that means is that you can be sleepy and pass out but as the alcohol is processed by your liver, you're not only going to wake up, you are going to wake up in a bigger state of panic because your brain kind of realizes something isn't right and is increasing the intensity of the signals that it is sending to compensate for that alcohol."[50]

4. **Get some exercise during the day, but not too close to bedtime**—I find exercise in the evening keeps my highly sensitive brain buzzing for too long and I find it difficult to calm down and get to sleep. I find working out in the morning is a great time because that is when I have the most energy and it helps me wind down at night.

5. **Empty your thoughts onto paper**—If you can't seem to shut your mind off when you lie down, keep paper and a pen close by to write things down. This will get them out of your mind and allow you to sleep and revisit them when you wake up. If I was worrying about what I had to do or remember for the next day, I would immediately write it down. That way, I could

release it from my thoughts. Journaling or writing in a diary can also be a good tool to get your thoughts out of your head and on paper. Leave those thoughts on paper until morning.

The Power of Distraction

During the day, it is easy to distract ourselves from negative thoughts or worry. But when we lie down at night, it can be the first time during the day that we can't escape them. Especially with anxiety, the amygdala, the part of the brain that senses danger, sends signals to the sympathetic nervous system telling it to get revved up. It might feel like you are ready to take action, although it is the time when you are supposed to be sleeping. This is very common with anxiety, but it can be very challenging to find ways to deal with it. Your body feels like it is reacting to a real threat, even if there is no real threat. It is like the amygdala is stuck on the "on" switch. Many times when this happens, we can feel helpless to stop it. The panic attacks I would experience at night as a young mom felt very real and very scary. It meant my heart was racing, my breathing was fast and shallow, and it would increase my blood pressure. If there was a real threat that I had to respond to, these things might have helped me, but they were not helping me sleep when I needed it most.

To distract yourself from a panic attack or if you are lying in bed and unable to calm yourself, the best tool for me was to get up and move my body until it calmed down but that can take a lot of time. Something as simple as breathing exercises, a bath, reading a book, or listening to some music can help to distract you from thinking about whatever thoughts triggered your response, or even to distract from the physical symptoms of a panic attack which can feel awful. Meditation is another good tool, and I will touch more on that in chapter 12.

A bedtime routine that helps calm you will make a world of difference. Gentle yoga, a hot bath, or reading are great ones, but anything that calms you down will get you from wired to tired quicker and will mean you will get a better night of sleep. A good night's sleep is one of the most important things you can do to nourish your mental wellness. If you have tried all of these things and are still struggling to get sleep, talk to a healthcare professional for a sleep aid. While there are risks of using sleeping pills in the long term, short-term sleep aids, when we need it most, can help our body get the rest it needs to operate properly.

When your body doesn't get the sleep it requires, anxiety levels will increase, enthusiasm and energy will decrease, and controlling your thoughts can seem impossible. A wise Twitter user named Drew Monson offered some great advice about this, tweeting:"I made a new rule: Never trust how you feel about your entire life past 9pm."[51] Since reading this, I have adopted this in my own life. I've realized that thoughts are usually junk after 9 p.m., and even worse at 2 a.m. or any time that I am overtired. Our brain requires sleep to operate effectively and that's why it is such an important requirement of good mental health. When I find myself overtired and ruminating over thoughts that are obviously junk, I tell myself to put those thoughts away, shut them off, and go get some sleep.

Making sure we are meeting our physiological needs at the bottom of Maslow's pyramid must come first! That means eating nutritious foods, staying hydrated, and getting enough sleep!

CUE "I SHOULD PROBABLY GO TO BED" BY DAN + SHAY

CHAPTER 8

The Third Shift:
What Working in the Media Industry and
Farming Taught Me about Self-Care

I recall hearing the F-word spoken for the first time ever and it came out of my mother's mouth! After taking supper to the field and getting home late, my mom had bathed and put my brother, my sister, and I to bed, surely exhausted from her day with three little ones under the age of ten in tow. I'm sure she was ready or already collapsing into her bed when my dad called out on our farm communication radio to bring something out to the field for him. I could tell how tired she was, but knowing Dad needed something urgently in the field, she woke us out of our beds, piled us in our pickup truck, and headed to the field. She was red in the face, mad as hell, and dropped the first F-bomb I had ever heard, expressing her displeasure in the situation. I didn't know the meaning of the word, but I knew it must be bad. I also knew how badly she felt in this moment. Suddenly, I felt badly for her too. I could feel her exhaustion and frustration like a shower of emotions, and as a child, I felt helpless to make it better for her, but I wanted so badly to protect her. I was a highly sensitive sponge, feeling that if I felt someone else's pain, I could make it my own and protect them. My mom was always a hard working and dedicated farmer, wife, and caretaker of all things, but I watched her try to do it all and many times work herself to exhaustion. I could see it. I could feel it. As a child, I remember thinking I would never be a farmer for this reason. While I felt a deep connection to nature, I was reluctant to help out on the farm because I attributed a lot of my hurt to what was supposed to be our family business. After all, it was almost always the reason we had to sacrifice something. My older sister Brandy had one hell of a passion for the farm. She would fight my brother to drive our 730 Case tractor with the stone picker behind. In contrast, my brother never had to fight. He was always given the opportunity to do any task on the farm and because of tradition and cultural norms was just expected to. I often watched them squabble over who would pick stones, drive grain truck, or work fields. I could see my sister's struggle, but I let her fight it alone. I didn't fight either one of them for my turn in the tractor. In my eyes, the farm stole precious time away from some of the most important relationships, and I didn't like that the farm took priority over almost everything else. My mom though, she was the best damn female farmer I knew. Her commitment, even through her exhaustion, was evident in everything she did. That night, that bad word in the pickup truck was simply a brief exposure of the struggles she endured on the farm as well. I knew farming was not for the faint of heart, and felt it wasn't right for my heart, but I also had the realization that I was more like my mother than I knew. The dirt under our fingernails connected us just as much as the blood running through our veins.

CUE "MOTHER'S DAUGHTER" BY MILEY CYRUS

Are you ready for another song?

Let's talk about work, baby
Let's talk about all the good things and the bad things it can be
Let's talk about work

If you aren't singing Salt-N-Pepa's *"Let's Talk About Sex,"* what generation are you from? It doesn't matter, keep reading. That song, or my version of it, was just for fun. They weren't talking about work in that song. They were talking about sex, something we will talk about later in this chapter, but first let's talk about work because that is something that is certain to get in the way of your mental wellness, and perhaps your sex life too!

Unless you are self-sufficient and live off the land, or have been handed a hefty inheritance, you likely need to work in some form or another. I've worked many different jobs, some involving physical labour when I worked maintenance at a local campground, other jobs I have worked behind a desk at a computer, and I've also served food at a local ski hill (yes, we have one of those on the prairies!) and an ice cream drive-in called Mr. Scoop alongside Highway 16. Work, in any form, is essential for us to put food on the table and a roof over our head. The thing with work is that some people choose a job because they love what they do, and they want to feel like going to work every day is fulfilling a desire, even if that job doesn't pay very well. While other people find a profession or job that pays really well but they may not like it very much or perhaps it doesn't fulfil any desire. Neither one of these are right or wrong and it is all based on your values and also your circumstance for what kind of work you choose.

If your value system is based on having more money than happiness, you might stay in a job you hate for your entire life, knowing that you will retire with a nice nest egg. If your value system is based on enjoying your work, and making enough money to live comfortably, then perhaps you are fine working at a job you love even though it doesn't pay that well. There is no right answer when it comes to work. Only you can decide which one is right for you.

If you are the kind of person who values purpose in your work, making you feel like you make a difference, or doing something you really enjoy, it is important to recognize that you are in a job that is fulfilling that desire. If you don't care, then work away and keep saving that nest egg!

I have learned that being in a job that I love is best for my mental health, however, that realization also came at a cost. When I was in high school and deciding what career path I wanted to choose, there were two choices I was entertaining: journalism and nursing. You might think those two things are so different from one another, but they really aren't in the sense of fulfilling a desire. Through every job I have had, even the first one in a video rental store at age thirteen, I've been eager to help other people. From finding the right video, or selling them a jug of milk, I can say that I held customer service and helping people very high on my priority list. It is perhaps why I appreciate good customer service to this day. Don't you love when a human answers the phone at a place of business? (I can't stand talking to a robot!)

I finished high school and I decided I wanted to take journalism because I loved to write, it had become such an outlet to get words and emotions down on paper. Writing had quickly become my superpower. I applied at a couple of Canadian universities. I got accepted into the pre-journalism program at the University of Regina. The two-year arts program was a prerequisite to apply to the School of Journalism, which was another two years. I completed my pre-journalism. I even took a couple extra courses that weren't required: an extra math and an extra French class because why the hell not? Keep in mind, I am a perfection-ist, a workaholic, and an Enneagram One. (This is a personality classification and Enneagram One personality means that we are often rigid workaholics and perfectionists who will suppress emotional needs in order to get things done.) Living only on a government-funded student loan, I was also making sure that I was maximizing every dollar I was going to spend. If I was going into debt to get a post-secondary education, I was going to make sure I maximized every dollar. I even did an exchange program and studied in York, England, for one semester because it was an opportunity to travel while getting my credits. I did everything I could to get into the School of Journalism. I crushed the interview (or so I thought). The School of Journalism only accepts twenty-six students each year. The number of students applying to the pre-journalism program was well over 200. That meant that I had less than a 15% chance of getting in. I was conditioned to know that if I worked hard, I would usually achieve whatever goal I was striving for. But for the first time, and during what I viewed as a major life goal, my effort and my attitude didn't matter. I didn't get in. There was nothing more I could do. The only choice was to surrender to a piece of paper that said I wasn't going to be a journalist. I had imagined my life graduating from the U of R with a degree in hand and a cushy CBC job lined up when I was done. Now, it seemed, I was surrendering. I had no control, something I worked so hard at for years to keep the environment around me safe and happy.

It was crushing. I was so disappointed. I spent two years preparing for this and then I couldn't do anything to change it. I could wait until next year and apply again, I could change career paths, or I could move to a community college and take an alternative program called media production. It was more of a hands-on program, teaching the technical and production side of media in addition to the writing aspect, which I was already mastering. I knew the program would complement the writing skills I already possessed, but I had concerns about going to a community college. My high school had always pushed universities over colleges and I couldn't help but feel I was taking a step down to go to a community college instead of a university. Was I ever wrong! When I relinquished control over the trajectory of my life and surrendered to alternatives, I realized it usually led me in the best places.

I applied to the Assiniboine Community College and got accepted into the program right away. (I crushed that interview as well.) I packed up and moved back to Manitoba's second largest city, Brandon, that is often called "the Wheat City" as it is surrounded by wheat fields. However, the Big Small Town, as I like to call it, is really home to the best 48,000 people around. I loved the community. When you see Manitoba license plates that say *Friendly Manitoba* on the bottom, they are surely talking about Brandon. I started the two-year program at Assiniboine Community College in the fall of 2002. It was such a change from university classes in auditoriums of 200 people, to a classroom of twenty-five. It was challenging and exciting, and we even broadcasted our own newscast Monday to Friday on the local cable channel. I loved every second of it. I loved my teachers, I loved the people I went to school with, and I loved the community of Brandon. When my program was complete, I applied for a practicum with Country Music Television (CMT) in Nashville, and my back-up choice was CKX television in Brandon (a small market CBC affiliate.)

My girlfriend Laura and I applied for our practicum at CMT together. We had plans to move to Nashville together and start our careers in the media industry while living in what we thought would be one of the greatest cities on earth while working at a place where country music and media met. We were pumped and ready to start the next phase of our life in the working world.

CUE PAUL BRANDT'S "SMALL TOWNS AND BIG DREAMS"

Laura got a letter inviting her to head south to Tennessee, but I did not. In my head, this practicum placement had felt so right. It felt like it was meant to be. I remember thinking, *Now what?* "I don't want to go without you," Laura said. My heart sank. Not only was I devastated, but I had ruined her plans as well. After surrendering, once again to circumstances, we both picked another placement in Manitoba. Laura was off to a TV station in Winnipeg, while I would stay in Brandon at a station whose key selling phrase was, "where local news comes first."

I remember my instructors at college telling me that CKX was such a great placement because it was small and I would be able to learn almost every job required to put together a newscast. I rolled my eyes. How could they possibly compare a national country music station to a small market CBC affiliate on the prairies? Turns out, they were right. I got the chance to do everything in the newsroom. I discovered something in that job. I discovered that people in the media industry are my kind of people. These are the people who go to work every day working under strict deadlines, tasked with telling other people's stories. It is fast-paced, competitive, and high stress. They are also willing to do this work, with hours that fluctuate, while getting next to nothing for a wage, and very often getting heckled by people about something that was reported or not reported, or how the weather forecast was wrong. But despite all of that, being a journalist gave me purpose in the best way. I was empathic in a way that made me perfect for telling other people's stories. I felt their stories with the strongest emotions, and I discovered that I was so good at it. I didn't just tell people's stories, I felt them. I was made for this job.

I was already employed by CKX working in master control (playing commercials) while attending college. During my practicum, I started reporting, then got the news anchor job for the noon-hour program, and eventually landed anchor for *CKX News at 6*, a one-hour local newscast that covered news from southwestern Manitoba. This was the station's flagship program. Farm families from across the region would come in the house in the evening and turn on this newscast. Almost everyone grew up with CKX around these parts, including me, as it was only one of three stations this area could get using the bunny ears on old tube TVs. I loved every second of my time there and had deep connections with everyone I worked with. The job was incredible. The pay was lack lustre, but the benefits were good, and the perks were even better. I was once given the opportunity to sky-dive in an interview I did to promote an upcoming air show in Brandon. I happily got strapped to a Canadian soldier and jumped out of a helicopter at ten thousand feet. Skydiving is incredible, because it allows you a chance to face an incredible fear in exchange for the best opportunity for joy imaginable. (Skydiving was one of the most peaceful, beautiful, and incredible experiences I've ever had and I would do it again in a hot minute.) But even the love for my job as a journalist couldn't stop me from going to a place where my mental health would suffer. Let me remind you that I was a perfectionist and a workaholic. I would immerse myself in my work because I loved it and would do it at the expense of my mental health. Remember that Enneagram One personalities are perfectionists that suppress their own emotional needs to get things done. I am an ideal employee in that sense. I would strive to never disappoint an employer. I was settling back into my old ways. My thoughts returning to my time as a young, depressed preteen when I thought if I could keep everyone happy around me, surely that would make me happy. Control, I thought, was the key. My work ethic was second to none and I was willing to prove that at the expense of anything. Eventually, it came at a cost. After just a couple years, I was burnt out, strung out, and having a hard time dealing with the fast-paced stressors of working in a newsroom, the very thing that I loved about the job.

I knew, very clearly, when it was time for me to leave CKX. It was a difficult departure. I was mentally exhausted. At the same time, I had fallen in love with my boyfriend of two years, James, a handsome hard-working farm boy with Ukrainian heritage who was farming two hours away from Brandon, in a mostly Ukrainian community twenty minutes east of where I grew up. His farm was just a few miles south of Riding Mountain National Park, a 3000-square-kilometre island of rugged forest, that is surrounded by a sea of farmland. I would learn after living here, that the higher elevation would be a challenging place to farm, one that would bring frosts late in the spring and early in the fall and heavier-than-normal precipitation that would keep heavy clay laden soil soggy longer than most other locations. Farming wasn't something that would allow James to move to Brandon (although he did for one winter and took a job welding so we could be together). Instead, he was forced to carry a heavy load of responsibility following his dad's departure from his life one day. He was already a few years invested into trying to save his family farm from foreclosure after his dad left both their family and the farm in a deteriorating state. James was doing his absolute best (and then some) alongside his mom, sister, and nephew, who for a while, all lived under one roof while we were dating. His passion for his family and the farm was evident in everything he did. I could see that, he too, was not handed an easy past, but his resilience was inspiring. He could fix anything with scraps from around the yard and only a few tools. Just like my grandpa taught us, nothing ever went to waste on the farm. Almost everything could be reused for something. James had the same no-waste philosophy of my grandpa who was a Depression-era farmer, but with the skills of *MacGyver (a resourceful character from a 1980's TV series)*. I often call James by the TV character's name when he is fixing something that seems unfixable just as the character on the TV series often did. But his task to turn a struggling farm into a successful one, was much bigger than those of the TV star's fictional emergencies.

At the age of twenty-five, I found myself contemplating a life on the farm alongside James. I knew if I chose to be with him, we had to commit to this life together, one that saw me moving to his farm, with the wounds of our past in tow, and commit to the life of a farmer. It meant a lot of sacrifice on my end, and I swore to myself I would never do that. I was hell bent on never being a farmer, but was considering it now. I had already lived in a little house on a paved street only miles from Manitoba farms, but it already seemed like a world away from living on one. That separation is perhaps what silences the agriculture industry's cries for help or blocks the attention of urban consumers on important topics. I had no misconceptions of what a move back to the farm meant for my future as I watched my parents work the dirt, reliving my mother's frustration years earlier in our blue GMC pickup. Farming is a humble existence. Farmers are often invisible when it comes to politics, media, and pop culture. It is a profession where you are tasked with feeding the world, with little to no credit in doing so, are often criticized for rising food prices or the way food is grown, all while the profession breeds burnout in isolation with little mental health supports.

I knew all of this, but farming was in my blood. It was the familiar feeling of the ground under my feet, dirt under my fingernails, no pavement in sight, and endless sunrises and sunsets that could turn a rotten day into a beautiful one with just a few moments of quiet reflection and slow relaxing breaths. In contemplating the decision, I remembered fondly of riding in the grain truck with my mom at harvest time during many late nights while Patty Loveless played on a staticky radio station and the grain dust hung in the night sky over one of those gorgeous sunsets. I acquired a love and appreciation for the farm life, but I was no stranger to what kind of commitment it was either. The sacrifices that came with the lifestyle were not lost on me, and I still had the invisible scars to prove it, in addition to student loan debt that I would be bringing back with me to the farm that I still hadn't paid off during my time at CKX.

I recently watched season three of the hit Paramount series *Yellowstone*. The overdramatized portrayal of ranching life has the patriarch John Dutton talking to his grandson Tait and he explains this in the most concise way. As the ranch owner complains to his grandson, saying, "Ranching is a terrible business," he goes on to list all the obstacles that ranchers must face. The list is a mile long, citing unpredictable prices and expense costs that are out of rancher's hands, government regulations, consumers complaining about how their food is produced, drought, losses due to predators, and more. His grandson replies with, "If ranching is so hard, how come we do it?" To which John Dutton replies, "Because it is one hell of a life."[52] That juxtaposition is exactly what was calling me back to the farm.

Farm Life, Best life?

The decision to farm with James was one that I knew meant I would have to be all-in just like my mom was on our farm. I wondered if I could do that. I remember the sacrifices growing up on the farm: missing school dances because it was harvest time, or not attending a family wedding because it was during seeding. I knew the lifestyle wasn't a forgiving one, by any means, but I also knew, for my mental health, that I couldn't stay in my current job long term, and I knew I loved James in a way I hadn't experienced before and he loved me hard right back. *Perhaps it would be different*, I thought. *Perhaps, I could make it different.*

I knew I needed to make a change, but the decision to leave CKX was one of the most difficult of my life. It was heart breaking to leave a place that felt like home. It was a job I was made for. I was good at it. I loved it. In the fall of 2007, I made the decision to pack up and leave Brandon in order to start my life together near Angusville with James, because I knew I simply couldn't be away from him.

CUE "ANYWHERE WITH YOU" BY JAKE OWEN

A year later, in my second-hand wedding dress I found in a classified ad (because I was and still am thrifty as hell and refuse to spend thousands of dollars on a damn dress!), we were married in front of 300 of our closest friends and family in a very big, small-town wedding kind of way with a live band, homemade food, and a cake made by one of my high school friends. Suddenly, I was a farmer. I was taking a job out of circumstance. It wasn't just a job; it was a role in a family farm and a family that also struggled with communicating their feelings effectively but thankfully did know how to show me unconditional love even if they couldn't speak the words. I knew the journey I was taking was going to be vastly different from the journey I had previously chosen for myself and worked so hard for. I had lost control again, but this time I surrendered willingly. I surrendered out of love for my husband, the desire to build a life together, and the gut feeling that surrendering in the past had led me to great things and this was likely to be no different. I knew life on the farm could be gorgeous, rewarding, and as John Dutton's character says, "One hell of a life." I needed to embrace it with a different mindset this time around and take on my new role as a farmer in a way that put my mental health first. I was willing to embrace the change, despite my contrasting feelings about it, and surrendered for my mental health, knowing that media held a very special place in my heart, but that farming was a familiar lifestyle for me. I knew my role on this farm would be very different than where I grew up, because I was investing my life here. I knew I could trust James to walk beside me through whatever was coming next. I knew I was better able to take on anything with an ally like him at my side, and I decided we would farm together for better or for worse, hoping that my worst was behind me.

CUE "NEVER TIL NOW" BY ASHLEY COOKE, BRETT YOUNG

Do you want to talk about stressors in farming? Where should I begin? Stressors in the agriculture industry are unique. Market fluctuations affect the price we get for our crops and livestock, we have very little control over input costs, weather is out of our hands, and there are some consumers who think we are trying to kill them using GMOs and chemicals, while some governments try to regulate an industry that they very clearly do not fully understand. Add to that, a workload that never ends (just changes with the seasons), isolation, and the stressors in the agriculture sector can be debilitating. If that weren't enough, compound all those things with a culture that leaves no room for vulnerability and the result is high rates of mental illness. According to a national survey by the University of Guelph, farmers face a greater level of stress, anxiety, depression, and risk of overall burnout than that of any other Canadian demographic. The survey's conclusions, "highlight a significant public health concern amongst farmers, and illustrate a critical need for research and interventions related to farmer mental health." It goes on to say that, "Scores for stress, anxiety, and depressions were higher, and resilience lower, than reported normative data. Females scored less favorably on all mental health outcomes studied, highlighting important gender disparities."[53] Sarah Smarsh writes about the economic inequality farmers, females, and lower-income groups face in her book *Heartland: A Memoir of Working Hard and Being Broke in the Richest Country on Earth*. Her experiences growing up in Kansas tell the story of how inequality and class can be a contributor to poor mental health in these populations when decision makers in government are unaware or uneducated about common problems. "Economic inequality is one cultural divide that causes us to see one another as stereotypes," she writes, "some of which allow the powerful to make harmful decisions in policy and politics."[54]

Did leaving my job in media and turning to farming heal my anxiety and depression? No. I can tell you it did not. In fact, it presented a whole new set of familiar challenges. I may have taken on a different career, with a different form of stressors, but stressors will find you everywhere: in any profession, or any situation, and especially in a society that tells us our worth is connected to our work, our weight, or our net worth. If we don't have a clear vision of why we are worthy without those things, we are always striving for something that doesn't have an end game. It is elusive. If you are looking for a low-stress place to live and work, you might want to pick Hawaii though. I recent study revealed that of all the US states, the life expectancy is highest in Hawaii. Dan Witters, Research Director of the Gallup National Health and Well-Being Index, wasn't surprised citing priorities in the Aloha state that includes "enjoyment, smiling, laughter, and happiness ... And stress is very low."[55] Obviously we can't all live in Hawaii, so finding that peace in our current profession, location, or economic class may be a challenge, but shouldn't be unattainable.

What I have learnt about working in media and agriculture is this: your mental health must be more important than your productivity. Without your mental health, there is no productivity. We are worthy of unconditional love regardless of our productivity, especially from ourselves.

What does this mean to our life? Be careful where you spend your time. Make sure it is serving your mental health. If what you're currently doing isn't working, try something else. I left a job I absolutely adored because it wasn't serving my mental health. I see now, it wasn't the job. I can overwork myself in farming the same way I was doing at CKX. I can experience the same burnout if I am not intentional about being proactive in taking care of my mental health. Weigh your options carefully when it comes to time management. Time, it seems, is another hot commodity when it comes to mental health. If we don't make time for our wellness, we will be forced to make time for our illness. I'm sure you have heard that before, but it holds more weight in your mental health than any other aspect of your well-being. Wellness coach Christa Lovas offered me some of the best advice about this. She says the best way to manage that to-do list when it feels overwhelming is to "do, delete, or delegate until it feels manageable."

Women who live and work on the farm can be susceptible to the third shift. The third shift is a phenomenon where women engage in off-farm employment, on-farm labour, and also take on responsibilities in the home. And some add volunteering in their community to that list as well. Sometimes, off-farm income is essential if money is tight and working on the farm is essential to keep the farm afloat, and when there are children to raise, there is inevitably laundry to do, and meals to make as the responsibilities on the home front are non-negotiable for moms (and dads). I used to work off the farm, but after having our kids, we decided I would stay home as my time on the farm paid more than the paycheque that came from town. On the farm, my tasks can include picking stones during seeding, running a combine during harvest, paying bills, doing farm books, crop planning, budgeting, running errands, preparing and delivering meals, driving kids to extra-curricular activities, and laundry, to name a few. (To be honest I could add a number of random tasks to that list on any given day.) My husband and I share a lot of responsibilities. Our roles are always changing with the seasons but there is no lack of demands from all directions. When somebody at the farm gets a flat tire, or my husband gets stuck in the field and needs to get pulled out, or one of my kids is home sick and needs extra care, things can change in my schedule quickly. Control is not something that is achievable for a perfectionist and highly sensitive person in this setting. It has been a battle. Every. Damn. Day.

The third shift can plague women in any profession, not just farming. I don't think it is just for women either, although I do think women are really good at taking on more and more responsibilities with an I-can-do-it-all attitude. When we attempt to do it all, and burnout ensues, we inevitably get to a point where we aren't any good to anyone, including ourselves. You know when you board a plane, and the crew says, "Put on your oxygen mask first before helping the person beside you?" That is the same kind of advice we all need to be reminded of discussing our mental health. We need to take care of ourselves first, before we can help others, or fully be present in our families, or in our jobs. We also have to remember the advice from Lovas: do, delete, or delegate, and adjust each of those accordingly depending on how much you feel you have the capacity to do.

It has taken many jobs and many years for me to realize that the only way for me to get time for my mental wellness routines (meal planning, exercising, reading, and yoga) is to do just that—create a routine. Making a daily schedule is the only thing that has worked otherwise those things are the first to go when time gets tight. You might feel like taking the steps and scheduling in the time to take care of your mental health seems impossible. I'm not going to lie to you, some days it is. Work can be just one thing that gets in the way. Family obligations can be another. There are so many more. Perhaps you have filled your schedule with too many things and now you don't know where to fit it in. At first, you might need to eliminate some things to make room. However, I promise you, when you make time to include mental wellness routines into all of your days, your days will get so much better.

For me that means when the kids go to school, I first and foremost, get my workout in as soon as they are on the bus. My workout comes before anything else in my day. It doesn't have to be a workout, and it doesn't have to be in the morning. For you, it might be taking time to have a cup of tea and a visit with someone. It might mean reading in the evening. With my achieving personality, it is easy to start a task and put my mental health routines aside. I've learned that eventually, I will pay the price when my mental health takes a hit. You might be someone who can endure under all circumstances. Let me say this: just because you are built to endure doesn't mean you should have to. I think anyone who is made to endure might have the potential to be the most successful monetarily or when it comes to reaching a physical goal like running a marathon, but when it comes to successful mental health, the ability to stop yourself from enduring at all cost is much more powerful.

I'm great at preaching this but putting it into practice isn't always easy. I have to remind myself daily that taking time to look after my mental health is priority number one. I love making super long to-do lists of what I am doing tomorrow or for the week and many times they are so unrealistic. A superhero would never even accomplish everything on that list but for some reason, I feel like if I keep going I will get it done. At the end of the day, when I look at the list of the eight to ten things I wrote down, and then realize I have only accomplished two of them, I get super bummed. These expectations can be productive in getting tasks done, but counter-productive to my mental health if it makes me feel defeated. In customer service, people say under promise and over deliver. I think enforcing that in our own life is good for our mental health. Set the bar at a realistic level instead of hoping to climb a mountain every day. It is great to be an overachiever but not at the expense of your mental wellness.

Dr. Jenn Hardy does a great job of explaining this in what she calls "affordable self-care." Hardy is a psychologist based in Tennessee. She has an Instagram page where she posts photos of advice that are handwritten on Post-it notes. This is my language! Some people operate their lives with fancy planners or calendars. Not me. I operate my entire life using Post-it notes. They are on my fridge, on my kitchen counter, beside my bed, in my purse, and all over my computer and office walls. My brain works well when I see reminders that are handwritten on bright sticky squares of paper. Post-it notes are life! When I see her little reminders on Post-it notes, it speaks to me. It is unconventional at a time when everything online seems to be so pretty and perfect. Her method is so effective because I find it so authentic.

I love her idea of affordable self-care. One that really stuck with me said this:

"Affordable Self Care: Set more realistic expectations about how long things take to get done."[56]

I think my head exploded when I read that one. It is such a simple idea. If you struggle with high expectations of yourself, and struggle with the guilt of taking time for yourself, it speaks directly to that. We can and should nourish our mental health by scheduling realistic time into our schedule as a priority before anything else on our to-do list.

Self-care has become an important topic in the last few years, but it really exploded when COVID-19 hit and mental health took a hit. Self-care has been perceived as the cure for burnout too. Being burnt out is not a badge of honour, but our society has led us to believe that it is. Many people thought that self-care was a relaxing weekend away. While that is a great place to start, and a couple days away can relax you, the problem is that if you walk straight back into the environment that caused the burnout, it won't change anything.

Here's what I've learned: the only way to see change is to find a way to manage stressors on a daily basis. If you need to get a weekend away to feel stress free, then take one. But you should also look for ways to feel that way while you are in any environment whether you are at work or at home. You can't always get rid of the stressors throughout your day, but finding ways to manage them and changing your mindset on how you react to them will aid in your mental wellness. Maybe that means listening to music while you work, taking a break for a walk, but maybe it also means just penciling out more time for the tasks on your to-do list. Self-care doesn't look the same for everyone. It might mean getting a task done to the best of your ability for one person, and the next person, it might just mean getting it done so you know that it was taken care of. It might also mean asking for help. Some of the best things I have done for my mental health to lighten the load here on the farm is getting my mother-in-law to help with meals when we are in the field, hiring a nanny to help watch the kids when I am busy, and hiring a housekeeper to clean my house when I know I am unable to do it at busy times. Taking a few things off my plate can make a world of difference. It can lighten the physical load but can also lighten the mental load as well. For the farm women who are reading this:

sitting on the lawn mower undisturbed for a few hours with your headphones on, I mean, does it get any better than that? Wherever you find some calm, even if it is on the seat of a riding lawnmower cutting the five acres of lawn you have, go do it!

I also find a massage once a month is a super helpful way for me to look after my body and mind. It is right up there with nutrition, exercise, and sleep. The benefits of massage include reduced muscle tension, improved circulation, stimulation of the lymphatic system, and a reduction of stress hormones. I was lucky enough to be living with one of my best friends during my time at university who was studying massage therapy. I benefited from her homework and had more than one massage on the kitchen table! However, there was a time when I couldn't afford to have a massage once a month. That's where Dr. Jenn Hardy's advice on affordable self-care come into play. The best tools to improve your mental wellness don't need to cost anything. I am fortunate enough to be able to hire help when I need it, but that wasn't always the case. If financially that isn't an option for you, I want you to know that self-care does not have to cost money. You can trade house cleaning for cooking. Bartering with a friend works too!

I saw a mom on social media post something the other day that made me furious. It said something like: "Going for groceries isn't self-care. Stop saying it is!" *How dare she?* I thought. How dare she judge other moms for finding joy in one of the simplest things. Getting out of the house when my kids were small was one of the greatest things for my mental health. If I had a chance to go for groceries without two kids in tow, it would have been the best self-care at the time. The thing about self-care is that, by definition, it is defined by "self." It is in the title! Nobody can decide what self-care is for another person. Only you know what things are good for your mental health. It can be dictated by circumstances and even stages of the life you are in at the moment. If you are a stay-at-home mom and going for groceries is the only time that Dad or Grandma watches the kids and you can get an hour alone, while doing a task on your to-do list that needs to be done to keep everyone fed, then that is 100% self-care. Another mom may have read this woman's suggestion that grocery shopping wasn't self-care and second guessed her ideals. *Don't do it.* I'm here to tell you that only you can decide what self-care is for you. Don't let anyone else decide for you. Your only task is to make the time for it (whatever that is) every day. Maybe it is having sex with your partner or yourself. (Physical touch is a great way to release serotonin, even if it is just a hug!) Maybe it is reading. Maybe it is exercising. Maybe it is baking.

Maybe it is reading and cuddling with your kids every night before bed. It can be so many things. Consistency is the key to success in anything. Consistency is also the key to achieving mental wellness. Self-care is an essential tool that must be done consistently to improve mental health regardless of where you work, or your circumstances.

CUE "I LOVE MYSELF TODAY" BY BIF NAKED

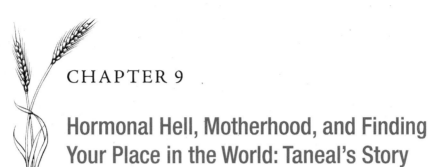

CHAPTER 9

Hormonal Hell, Motherhood, and Finding Your Place in the World: Taneal's Story

Hormones are crucial. They are in many ways the command centre of your body, including your mental state. As a preteen, the topsy turvy years of puberty and the beginning of my period led to a hormone imbalance, which contributed to my depression. My childbearing years were a goddamn rollercoaster with hormones and emotions, and now as I approach my forties, I continue trying to balance my hormones to keep my emotions in check.

Dr. Wendy Davis, ND, is an expert on women's health. She has worked as a naturopathic doctor for sixteen years. Her practice, Harmony Health Clinic, focuses on helping clients achieve total body wellness. Her approach is to listen to the concerns a patient has and helps them find the root of the problem and regain wellness and optimal health. She has a special interest in hormonal health for women and has spent much of her career studying the effects of women's hormones on their mood and well-being.

What she knows for absolute certain: stress is the number one cause of hormone imbalance. When a woman's body is under stress, the adrenal glands release cortisol, the primary stress hormone. According to the Mayo Clinic, "When cortisol is released, it increases our body's blood sugar levels, alters immune system responses, suppresses the digestive system, the reproductive system, and growth processes."[57] It can also wreak havoc on our ability to control mood, motivation, and fear. When we are under stress, it can also rob the body of its thyroid hormones, melatonin, estrogen, and progesterone.

Progesterone was the hormone that was being robbed from me when my kids were small and demands on the farm and in the home were overwhelming. Progesterone is a crucial hormone in a woman's body, especially for fertility and getting our bodies ready to implant an egg and grow a human. After you deliver that human, progesterone levels drop, and estrogen increases. This process helps to initiate milk production to feed that new baby you are now looking at, with wonder at how your body can produce such a sweet thing in only nine months.

A woman's regular cycle will include levels of progesterone that are low at the beginning of the cycle (when her period starts) and stay low throughout the follicular phase. Once ovulation takes place, progesterone levels increase during the second half of the cycle (the luteal phase), but if conception doesn't take place, progesterone will drop again before her period starts. However, if your body is low on progesterone or is robbed of progesterone because it is busy making the stress hormone, cortisol, that low level of progesterone will show up with symptoms that include headaches, migraines, anxiety, sleeplessness, depression, low energy, and a slow metabolism. (Spoiler alert: this can also happen during menopause!)

What does this mean for women who are super stressed and have high levels of cortisol? Dr. Davis explains how this can have an effect on the production of GABA, which is a calming neurotransmitter. "The body steals from making progesterone [and shifts] to making cortisol. When we have lower progesterone, we don't get GABA. It is a chemical cascade, and when we don't get GABA, we tend to be more anxious. It is like putting your foot on the gas pedal 24-7."

I think Dr. Davis' comparison to putting your foot on the gas pedal is a fair one to make for all women. Whether you are at home raising a family, or chasing career goals, or both, women are extremely good at multi-tasking. However, unless you are good at setting boundaries, piling too much on your plate can happen very quickly. And everyone's tolerance for how much stress they can handle depends on their current mental state. I've heard a saying that uses a great analogy for this: Maybe you think someone doesn't have a lot on their plate compared to you. But maybe their plate is smaller than yours and doesn't have a lot of room to begin with. Or maybe their plate is paper, and their flimsy paper plate can't hold as much as your sturdy ceramic plate can. Or maybe their plate was broken and is now held together with glue.

Whatever your plate is made of, get to know the load it can carry when you are healthy and feeling well. But also get to know the load it can carry when you are not feeling well, or feeling overly stressed or worried, or have a lack of sleep. That load will constantly be changing based on circumstances and how you are feeling. Unless we are acutely aware of how we are feeling, and really paying attention to how we respond, it can be easy to drop an overloaded plate.

The overload that I felt with my kids, and that many mothers experience, comes from a place of wanting to be a good mom for your kids, a good partner, and good at your day job. But that overload and desire to help everyone all the time can lead to losing yourself if self-awareness isn't practiced along the way. Author Doe Zantamata put it best: "When you try to make things better for a lot of people, you may end up making things worse for yourself. A little self-sacrifice is noble, but depriving yourself of too much will only leave you depleted."[58]

Who hasn't felt depleted when becoming a parent? If you are a mother or a father who has had to stay at home to parent small children, you will know what being isolated feels like. I have never felt loneliness like the time following the birth of my two children. When you come home with a newborn, everyone showers you will gifts and food and they want to give the baby attention and everyone passes it around. And you become this peacock like you are showing off your colourful feathers to the world. Like you want to announce, "Look what I made!" While it is a celebratory time, it can also be the calm before the storm. The storm of hormone changes, which can happen when you are alone with children, when your spouse goes back to work, or your extra help goes home, and you are left to learn how to parent alone. The storm starts brewing—cue stress and cortisol.

Taneal Semeniuk knows all too well about the storm called postpartum depression and has been very vocal about her experiences in hopes of helping other new moms recognize the signs that they might be experiencing it as well. The thirty-eight-year-old mom runs a support group called Mothers Helping Mothers in her community of Russell, Manitoba. The group provides a safe space for mothers to share and support each other through the challenges and joys of parenting. She has also hosted an event in her community by the same name that brought mental health professionals together and a place for others to share their experiences.

When Taneal had her first baby in February 2009 at twenty-seven, she felt prepared for what motherhood was going to throw at her. Going into her pregnancy in the best shape of her life, and after preparing alongside her husband Jared about what might come by doing prenatal classes with a mid-wife service, Taneal admits she had no idea what was coming. "The midwife went over information on labour and delivery, breast-feeding, and postpartum depression."[59] Taneal discounted the information she was being given on postpartum depression. "I totally phased out," she says, "because I literally thought that [information] was only for the weak." She couldn't have expected what would happen when it was time to give birth. "I had a solid mindset that it wouldn't happen to me."

After a late night of watching TV with her husband, Taneal went into labour around 4:00 a.m. The couple, staying at her parent's place, had to stop at home for a bag, stop for gas, and then embark on a two-hour drive to the hospital in Brandon where she was going to deliver. Before delivery, Taneal walked the halls of the maternity ward, lined with pictures of smiling babies, and remembers thinking how excited she was to finally get to hold her baby in her arms.

After a traumatic delivery with postpartum hemorrhaging, where she lost a lot of blood and her body went into shock, the situation quickly became life-threatening. The midwife handed off the crying (and healthy) baby girl to a nurse to get examined, and then immediately turned her attention back to Taneal. She remembers the midwife's tone changing very quickly. Taneal knew something was wrong. She remembers thinking, *Is this the way I am going to die?* and asking her husband, "Am I going to be OK?" After the doctor got the bleeding under control and the placenta delivered, Taneal was able to calm down and was in the midst of trying to process what just happened, but it was time to put her focus on the baby.

"I tried to put my hair in a ponytail and I couldn't even lift my arms. Then they handed me the baby and I didn't have the strength to hold her. All I wanted to do afterwards was sleep and shut down and rest and heal." But she quickly discovered that the new reality didn't involve any of that. The next few hours and days turned into feeding baby, changing baby, checking stitches from her episiotomy. If you are unfamiliar with this term, it is when a woman's vagina rips or is cut between the vagina and the rectum to allow the baby to be delivered. Taneal spent five days in the hospital, where she used a breast pump throughout the day struggling to get her milk to come in. Her nipples were chapped and bruised from pumping and trying to get the baby to latch onto her breast to start breastfeeding. She was exhausted, everything was hurting, and she remembers telling her husband on day three, "I just want to go home with you, me, and the dogs."

The midwife, recognizing Taneal's lack of bonding with her new baby, knew something wasn't right and after being sent home from the hospital, set up weekly visits with her family doctor. She also made sure the community's public health nurse would pay a visit as soon as they got home. Taneal's husband Jared was off work for three weeks so they could all adjust to being a family of three.

After doing a thorough questioning of the new mom, and Taneal being honest about how she was feeling, the public health nurse recommended a group in the community that was funded by Provincial Health called Baby Steps. The group took place at a local church basement where moms (and some dads) would meet to talk about a different topic every week. It was also a time to share parenting stories with each other. At a time when all of Taneal's friends were people she worked with, and most still single or without babies in tow, the group served an important place for her to make connections. "All I wanted to do was have the life that I had previous to having this baby come out of my body and getting up every two hours to feed it. I just wanted my old life back, and not have to deal with this thing that took everything away from me." Taneal recalls sitting at Baby Steps and watching one mom, whose baby started crying, and the mom knew exactly what to do. Taneal asked her, "How do you know what to do?" The mom replied, "I fed him a little while ago, so chances are he is hungry or needs a change. I'll try both first. Chances are they don't cry for unknown reasons."

Taneal realized she had to change the narrative in her head for the sake of her baby. "I didn't know why my baby was crying...I was so checked out...I remember sitting on the couch, my baby was still in her pyjamas from the night before, I didn't brush my hair or teeth before I left the house. I couldn't hide it. All I could do was sit there and cry."

Taneal took advantage of all the help that was available to her, except one. Medication. Her doctor recommended an anti-depressant. He gave her three different options to explore. Because breast feeding was a priority, Taneal's midwife had concerns with two of the medications passing through the breast milk and concluded that there was really only one option she would consider while breastfeeding. Taneal says after researching the side effects of the antidepressant, she still wasn't comfortable taking it, naming side effects such as insomnia, weight loss/weight gain, and lack of appetite, which were all things she was currently experiencing.

Taneal believes medication likely would have made a difference in her recovery had she been more willing to embrace it. Years later, she knows that when she is in a bad place, she is prepared to take medication knowing that it is an option. At the time though, she declined.

When Jared went back to work after three weeks, she knew her anxiety was unmanageable. If she wasn't getting sleep because of feeding the baby, she would lie in bed consumed with guilt about not being able to walk their two dogs, or not being able to vacuum the floor of the house— worrying about anything and everything at 4:00 a.m. Her brain wouldn't stop. She was experiencing a constant flow of adrenaline. "I knew I was not well, but I still didn't want to be a statistic on medication. I was barely functioning. I felt a lot of shame in taking medication." She knows now that there is no shame in finding help, whatever that looks like. One day, when she was alone with the baby, sleep deprived and feeling exhausted, she called Jared at work and told him to come home. "I don't trust myself to not harm the baby," she told him. "I was a donkey on the ledge," she recalls.

From that point on, Taneal had family members stay with her as much as possible, and then opted to move in with her parents during the week while Jared was at work to get help looking after the baby. Taneal tried journaling at night to free up space in her mind, she was taking more breaks, getting more sleep, and started taking vitamins B and D through the advice of a naturopath. As the weeks went on, things started to get better. Spring was starting to take shape in Manitoba and "getting outside made a huge difference," she said. She also attributes a lot of her recovery to the realization that two of her aunts suffered postpartum depression—one of them suffering psychosis, where she heard voices and wanted to harm her child. She says hearing their story helped her to realize that the things she was experiencing wasn't so abnormal, even for some of her family members. While the knowledge that she may have been genetically pre-disposed to postpartum depression may have helped her journey, just knowing someone else who was close to her experienced mental health issues was a sort of healing as well.

Taneal realized that she was overthinking something as simple as just leaving the baby to go outside. She was consumed with worry about whether or not the baby would have to eat while she was outside, convinced that her role as a mother meant staying beside her baby every waking minute. Her mother demanded that Taneal go get some fresh air while she watched the baby. Her brother took her out on the quad to go sit with the cows and he asked her, "Do you see that mother cow over there?" She had just had a calf a few days earlier and was standing there nursing. He said, "How do you think that mother cow is feeling right now?" The conversation about nature and how trusting the process of motherhood stuck with her. Taneal says she had days where she would sit and look out the window and cry, just wishing for it to go away. Eventually, it did get better, but not without weeks of struggling to feel like she didn't fit the mom role she was supposed to be in. She attributes the level head of her husband who reassured her that it didn't matter if she nursed, or didn't, or walked the dogs, or didn't. He was constantly reassuring her as a mom that she had nothing to prove and that they were going to do whatever was right for their family. Taneal admits that the whole experience, "wasn't easy for him." But she is thankful that he helped her to let go of any expectations she had about what kind of a mom she thought she was supposed to be. She was ready to let go of the guilt and be whatever mom she could be for her baby.

Dr. Wendy Davis says there is a hormonal reason moms feel down after childbirth. "When women are pregnant, a lot of the hormones are super high, and then within the first day or two postpartum is when there is a huge drop." A drop in progesterone can wreak havoc on a new mom, she says. "Typically, during the majority of pregnancy, progesterone, which is a feel-good hormone, is really high." Progesterone is one of the hormones that makes ligaments elastic, making women's bodies able to stretch and accommodate a growing baby. "But it is also why a lot of women have that euphoric feeling," she says. Referring to why some new moms explain that they feel a connection with their baby the minute it is born. "They just feel wonderful and that's just because progesterone stimulates GABA, which is a relaxing neurotransmitter." She explains why a mom's mood can also change very dramatically and very quickly after childbirth. "Progesterone is also given off by the placenta, so when there is no more need for the placenta, or there is no more placenta, progesterone drops and that's when a lot of the mood really changes." Dr. Davis says it is normal for a woman to feel down but adds, "for some women, if there is increased stress levels, then our natural adrenaline production of progesterone goes down and that's when we tend to get a little more of the mood issues, depression, and unable to cope."

Dr. Davis tells new moms that it is important to find support wherever they can, if they find themselves struggling. "In addition to the low progesterone, we also get the constant sleep deprivation that increases cortisol and cortisol is the main stress hormone." Because cortisol will rob the body of progesterone, the only way to replenish it is to decrease stress on the mom. "Anything she can do to reduce cortisol levels, so that would be things like a cat nap during the day and different supplements would help." Dr. Davis recommends supplements that are safe for mom and babies, and will offer adrenal support to reduce cortisol. This might also help the baby be less anxious too. "Your baby is going to be getting that cortisol from the breast milk as well. If mom is anxious, then baby will likely be anxious too."

Dr. Davis recommends herbal supplements, like passionflower, that can be as easy as making a cup of tea with it or taken in a capsule form.

She adds that diet plays a huge roll as well, explaining how increased blood sugar levels can increase cortisol. "Be mindful with your food. Keeping blood sugar levels stable is really crucial because when we are tired, we tend to crave sugar a little bit more and when we eat too much sugar, our blood sugar levels yo-yo and our moods yo-yo so it can lead to a lot more anxiety and depression." While Dr. Davis recognizes that new moms can't always get the rest they need, they can control the nutrition their body needs, recommending snacks that include fat and protein consistently. Things like eggs, apples, and nut butter. "Simple sugars like a piece of toast, handful of crackers, or a banana will get blood sugars up quickly but they crash quickly so you need to have foods that take a little bit of time to get into your bloodstream but then stay in your bloodstream longer. They take longer to metabolize."

Taneal remembers when things got better and she felt less stressed as a new mom, she would get excited about little things again like buying a new set of earrings, something she wouldn't have done weeks prior. When she went back home from her parents' house, she also made little goals for each day, helping to make a schedule, and having something to look forward to each day. She also realized, from the experience, that asking for help when she needed a break was one of the most important ways she was able to protect her mental wellness as a new mom.

CUE UP CARRIE UNDERWOOD'S SONG, "SMOKE BREAK"

This song is so good we are going to play it twice!

I don't recommend smoking or drinking for your mental wellness but this song clearly indicates the need and importance of getting a break and that's why I love it. As parents, we convince ourselves that we don't need a break. Let me assure you, we all need a break sometimes, and those breaks are what makes us better parents. While asking for help might be hard to do when struggling with mental health issues, it is imperative to ask for help when we need it. Remember that there is no prize handed out for struggling alone, but there are consequences.

Taneal and her husband had three more additions to their family: another girl and a set of twin girls, becoming a family of six. Taneal is well known in her community for providing support and resources for new moms and was recognized by the Province of Manitoba for her advocacy work.

Hormones can go awry for many reasons, not just following childbirth. Menopause, or an overactive or underactive thyroid, can cause things like estrogen dominance or a shortage of progesterone that can throw your hormones a curveball and ultimately your mood as well. If you are female and feeling unwell, hormone levels might be the first thing to investigate. There are tests available that can indicate where hormone levels are at, and supplementation can be added to address shortcomings. One test I found helpful is called the DUTCH test, which uses dry urine samples to measure hormone levels. There are also blood and saliva tests available to investigate hormones. Some other experts on fertility and hormone health that offer a lot of advice on the subject include Dr. Lara Briden, who has written books on the subject, as well as hormone specialist Dr. Mariza Snyder, who offers her advice through podcasts and books as well.

If you find your hormones are not balanced, Dr. Wendy Davis also suggests detoxification, recommending women eliminate certain household products, foods, and plastics in their homes in order to decrease artificial hormones that could be adding to the problem.

A note to all the tired mamas out there: It is OK to be short fused, overwhelmed, fed up, and tired. So tired. You are not alone. Asking for help is hard. Asking for help is humbling. It's OK to ask for help. I'm giving you permission. Your hormones need a reset, just like you need a reset, and asking for help or taking a break when you need it is the only way to rise up when you feel down.

CUE "RISE UP" BY ANDRA DAY

The COVID Connection

The amazing thing that happened during the COVID-19 pandemic outbreak around the world in 2020 was that people of all ages experienced degraded mental health similar to what new moms often experience after bringing a newborn home. People were told to stay at home in quarantine and to social distance themselves from others. The result was a society that was suddenly deprived of social interactions and connection, one of the most basic requirements of good mental health. The lack of these experiences left people feeling alone, anxious, and depressed.

Social media became an online community of people who were quarantined and posts on social media like, "And just like that, nobody ever asked a stay-at-home mom what she did all day" went viral. While the comparison made moms laugh all over the world, it suddenly shed light on the fact that mothers, at least in North America, for years have been in the same self-isolating situations. Left to feed a newborn every two hours, change diaper after diaper, and, for many of them, do it alone. I'm speaking about what happens in North America and perhaps this isn't the case in other areas of the world. Some tribes in Africa raise children with a dozen or more women to look after the little ones and babies in the group and that makes me wonder if perhaps we are doing it wrong. Support groups, like the one Taneal created, can and should play a very important role for new moms.

Here on the Canadian prairies, there are so many prenatal checkups when a woman is pregnant. But the mental health aspect postpartum is the piece of the puzzle that has traditionally been lacking in our health care here in Canada. The focus is almost always on the baby, measuring its weight and height to ensure growth. Very little is paid to the mom that is providing the necessity of life to that baby. Things are starting to shift in the last few years, but more emphasis needs to be put on mental wellness. Not only for new moms, but for every population. While mental wellness is starting to gain ground now, a whole lifestyle approach to health needs to transform our health care system, looking more at lifestyle changes and less on pharmaceuticals that simply mask the symptoms.

If there is something to be grateful for from the pandemic of 2020, it is that mental illness came to the forefront because so many people experienced it at the same time. For years, when new mothers were diagnosed with postpartum depression, it was a big label that nobody was willing to talk about. As we've discovered, hormones and stress can play a huge role. But how much is hormones and how much is isolation? It is just basic human nature to crave interaction and connection. When we don't have it, loneliness can lend itself to depression and anxiety. Dr. Gabor Maté wrote about the importance of social interactions to our health in his book, *When the Body Says No: The Cost of Hidden Stress*. He writes, "Interactions with other human beings—in particular, emotional interactions—affect our biological functioning in myriad and subtle ways almost every moment of our lives. They are important determinants of health."[60]

Another thing the global pandemic of COVID-19 taught us was that our governments don't actually know that much about mental health when it comes to giving people advice. Health care providers and government leaders in big cities like London and Paris were telling people to stay inside their homes. They were told not to go outside. We watched the news as police officers in Hyde Park were riding horseback with batons in hand, threatening people to get out of the park for sunbathing or face consequences. In an attempt to keep people healthy from the looming threat of the virus, what they were actually doing was suppressing their immune systems and compromising their ability to fight off the virus.

You may think, *How were they suppressing their immune system?* Very simply, mental health plays a huge role in how you feel and affects your overall physical health. Ever notice how you get a cold or a flu easily when you are run-down? Your body's immune system can work more efficiently when you are mentally (and physically) at your best. There is a saying that we are all just complicated house plants because we all need water and sunshine, the only difference is that we have complicated emotions. While that may seem like a funny little joke, there is truth there. We do need sunshine. Every day. We aren't going to die without sunshine every day, but our mental health will suffer. Even my eleven-year-old daughter Ava, who just experienced a long Manitoba winter, knows how important it is. On the first day of spring, she said to me, "Mom, why do we feel so lazy in the winter and when spring comes, we seem to have so much more energy? Where does that energy come from?" My first thought was: *She is so self-aware! Impressive, this will serve her in life.* Then I replied with, "The sun. It comes from the sun." My second thought was: How can we harness that energy for winter and counter sluggish feelings? The answer might be vitamin D supplementation and, more importantly, absorption.

There has been abundant research that states vitamin D is an important supplement for mental wellness. The best kind is from the sun, but we can't always get enough if we are demographically challenged. While there are varying recommendations, a daily dose of around 400 to 1000 IU is where most recommendations start and go up from there. Being someone who has battled both depression and anxiety, I can tell you that number is not nearly large enough. If you live in Canada, Dr. Davis says that our vitamin D supplementation should be much higher. In the winter months, I take around 5000 IU per day and supplement my vitamin D (paired with vitamin K2 for calcium absorption) with a HappyLight in my office that provides artificial light when I can't get enough outside in the winter months. If you aren't demographically challenged like us in Manitoba and live in Hawaii or another part of the world with adequate sunshine, rest assured, you are likely getting enough.

While vitamin D might play a role, our exposure to the sun might be far more important to our serotonin levels. A few sessions in a tanning bed each winter has been an absolute saviour for me and that is where I get the most bang for my buck when it comes to sunshine supplementation. I know the Canadian Cancer Society is going to see this and want to chase me down and scold me, but just hear me out. We know that tanning beds can cause skin cancer. Research has shown that when your skin is exposed to UV rays from the sun, tanning beds, or sun lamps, you may be at greater risk of getting skin cancer. But some studies have also found a link between low vitamin D levels and cancer risk and progression.[61] It is my opinion (and only my opinion) that if you think anxiety or depression is a serious risk to your health (and perhaps your life), tanning might far outweigh the risks of getting skin cancer. I believe this to be true for myself, but perhaps not for everyone. Tanning for just ten to fifteen minutes two to three times a week can drastically affect my mood.

Not likely in Canada in the winter, but in other places around the world, one hour in the sun can provide up to 40,000 units of vitamin D. So telling people in large cities to stay inside is unfathomable to me when it comes to taking care of their mental health and, in turn, their immune systems. Our connection to outside, fresh air, and nature is something that our bodies were made to crave. The sunshine requirement is essential. Someone who struggles with mental health should be outside for a minimum of thirty to forty-five minutes per day.

So, what did COVID-19 teach us? It taught people more about the importance of mental health than ever before and all the tools we need to nourish it, including getting outside every single day. The other lesson we learned was the importance of connection, something I would argue is one of the most important components to good mental health.

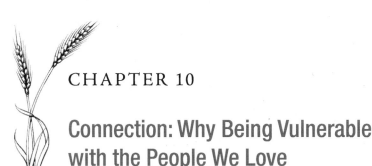

CHAPTER 10

Connection: Why Being Vulnerable with the People We Love Nourishes Our Mental Health

"Connection is the energy that exists between people when they feel seen, heard, and valued; when they can give and receive without judgement; and when they derive sustenance and strength from the relationship."— Dr. Brené Brown[62]

I start this chapter with a quote from Dr. Brené Brown's book *The Gifts of Imperfection* because I think her research on shame and vulnerability is so valuable. If you haven't read her books, listened to her TED talks, or heard her podcasts, please put them at the top of your to-do list. She is phenomenal and in alignment with the beliefs I hold about honouring our mental wellness through vulnerability and being authentic. If I didn't hold value in being authentic and vulnerable, I wouldn't be writing this book and giving every detail of my life to share with you. I truly believe that our vulnerabilities need to be shared to build meaningful connections.

Social stimulation has been found to be very important for brain health. Finding someone you can connect with at an emotional level, someone who you are able to share your thoughts and emotions with, and how you process your thoughts and emotions are critical for everyone, but especially for people who struggle with anxiety and depression. Connection identifies our commonalities, our differences, and supports our mental health in times of vulnerability. It is essential for emotional health and, in turn, our mental health.

Just as love and affection are essential to a child's healthy brain development, adults also need those connections to navigate life properly. In a world that values dollars instead of relationships, we are often found chatting with robots online, using self checkouts, and sacrificing those essential connections at every turn.

Now, more than ever, we must seek out and cultivate reconnection in a world that is fostering habits on how to disconnect from other humans.

While our online lives might be filling a need for connection using social media, the good stuff can't be substituted: the handshakes, the eye contact, the exchange of smiles, and most importantly, conversations with each other. We need one another in life to be happy. We also need one another to help us through the tough stuff. We need friends and family who act as life rafts, keeping us afloat when we feel like drowning. We need people who will jump right into the water beside us and swim us back to shore. You know the people I am talking about? They are the ones who would stop anything at any time if you needed them. We need these people just about as much as we need air to breathe. Whether it is a classmate, a co-worker, friend or a spouse.

For women, finding connections in the ag world can be as difficult as securing credit and access to land. It seems women in the agricultural world are still facing gender specific obstacles. So many times, I've stood beside James in front of someone we do business with, and have been completely ignored even though we both make decisions about the land we farm, how we sell our crop, and the daily details of our operation. I get tired of trying to prove myself. Gender specific barriers in farming is something that can be a roadblock when it comes to making connections in our industry.

It is from those experiences that I'm really good at thinking I don't need to rely on anyone, with a belief that needing someone might make me weak or vulnerable, but the truth is we can be independent and still require connection, and that doesn't make us weak. As Brown's research has shown, when you are vulnerable with others, the reward is connection. When we embrace those uncomfortable feelings and talk about difficult things, it connects us in a way that feeds our soul. In contrast, when we forget to be vulnerable with the people who we care about the most, it can have devastating consequences, leading to a break in a friendship and ending in divorce when it happens in a marriage. Connection is crucial in relationships and is a requirement for good mental health.

I often have to remind myself to keep being open and honest with James about how I am feeling, and remind myself to give him support when he needs it too. At the end of a long day, I just want to crawl into bed and cocoon, but that is usually when he wants to talk. I've had to make a conscious effort to stay connected for a few minutes before bed knowing that is the time of day he wants to connect. I'm a morning person and often my time to have conversations is when I first get out of bed. When one spouse or partner doesn't want to burden the other with their needs or is scared to ask for what they need in a relationship, it is an absolute killer of connection. Let me say it again. It is an absolute killer! The fear that their needs might inconvenience the other person, or their requests might hurt the other spouse, can lead to a lack of connection over time and ultimately the death of any previously established connection.

This has played out in my own marriage. Together, my husband James and I make a great team on the farm. We are fantastic business partners. We are sounding boards for each other about every decision. We are really good at exploring all our options, questioning and challenging each other, and trying new things, seeing what works and what doesn't work, and learning from others about how to do things better. We have also been really good at investing our money in places that will show return. Good business partners? Check! We got that down. We are also really great parents, aligning our values and raising our kids in a way that reflect those values. Good parents? Check! We got that down too (or at least we are trying). Dancing partners? Absolutely! I married a Ukrainian dancer, and there is nothing I love more than tearing up the dance floor to some country music, a seven-step or a heel-toe, and he is a phenomenal dancer. There is nothing that makes me happier than to be on the dance floor with my husband. It truly is magic. James and I really are meant to be in business and life together. We make an incredible team. We complement each other and call each other on our bullshit too. Together, I think we could take on almost any task, but that is if—and only if—we are being honest and vulnerable with each other and make the time for connection.

There was a time when our marriage went from fiery hot to mediocre because of a lack of connection. We were busy growing the farm, kids, and forgot to make time for each other. I've heard many couples experience the same thing at this phase in life. The phase I am talking about is when you have small kids, and you are building a family and career, and you are so laser focused on certain goals and assume your marriage will withstand it all. Let me tell you that it won't. What I have found to be true: marriage needs vulnerability to thrive. I'm not for one second saying that vulnerability will solve all relationship problems and while I know divorce happens for a myriad of reasons and some people are legit better off apart than together, I am simply speaking about what has worked for us. Being vulnerable with each other seems to be the key to staying connected in a marriage. That, and the advice of Gary Chapman. If you are married or in a relationship and haven't read Gary Chapman's book *The 5 Love Languages: The Secret to Love that Lasts*, please go read it now. After reading his book and taking the quiz together, I learned that my husband's love languages are physical touch and acts of service. James learned that mine are words of affirmation, and quality time. Chapman's book changed the way we show love for each other and, ultimately, is what keeps our connection strong. We always need a constant reminder to stay vulnerable with each other, and most marriages need that advice too as I've discovered through the advice of another small-town Manitoba girl and fellow author Ashleigh Renard.

If you like to read erotica and self-help books, Renard writes about her personal development journey in a memoir that encompasses both genres. Her book, *Swing*, is about her almost-affair with another man, after her and her husband embrace the swinger lifestyle but forget to embrace vulnerability in their relationship along the way. Most readers won't be able to relate to their racy sex life but will draw parallels in raising kids, growing careers, and feeling the demands of life. Renard found a man outside of their marriage who checked all the boxes of connection, as Brené Brown defines it: she was feeling seen, heard, and valued. She felt like she could give and receive without judgement. She developed the relationship out of a desire for connection, something she and her husband Manny were lacking after focusing on almost everything (and I mean everything) but their connection.

As it turns out, the relationship Renard was pursuing wasn't what she needed. In her realization, and after contemplating divorce and acknowledging her options, Renard discovers that embracing her own values and vulnerabilities with her husband was what she really needed to feel the connection that she was longing for, but it was going to take work. It always does. We need to cultivate those connections, or they degrade. She says contemplating divorce as an option—for so long avoiding the very thought of it—helped her realize what was best for her. "The reason that our marriage actually got better was because I let go of the idea that staying married was the best outcome. That is when things actually started to change."[63]

With the help of counselling, Ashleigh and Manny became aware of their own needs and the importance of communicating them with each other. "I'd learned that very few of the choices we made had the power to save or destroy us, but the fear of them did have the power to keep us each in a tiny little box," Renard writes. "A box that was not a natural and joyous fit for many of us, if it really fit anyone at all.

And that fear did have the power to keep me small, and scared and half alive."[64] She admits that "What started as a journey for excitement and connection uncovered that we had what we needed all along. We just had to allow it and uncover it."

Dr. Brené Brown says we don't have to be an open book with everyone, "Our stories are not meant for everyone. Hearing them is a privilege, and we should always ask ourselves this before we share: 'Who has earned the right to hear my story?'" She goes on to say, "We don't need love and belonging and story-catching from everyone in our lives, but we need it from at least one person."[65]

Being vulnerable with the people we care about, either our spouse, a family member, or a friend, has the most potential for deep meaningful connection. That connection will only exist if we are willing to be ourselves, ask for what we need, and tell each other how we feel without the fear of being judged. If we can do this, it will make way for some of the best relationships in our lives, something that is essential for our mental health.

Sometimes, it is hard to be vulnerable, especially if you feel you are being judged, criticized, or aren't being heard. I have a friend whose husband spends a lot of time working away from home, and she is often left with double the responsibilities when he is gone during the week. When he came home on a weekend, she told him that she was feeling overwhelmed, burnt out, and generally unwell. She was essentially waving a white flag and asking for help. When he dismissed her feelings, and didn't offer to change the status quo, she told me, "Why do I even bother?" This can be extremely frustrating, and no doubt, was disappointing. Even though she didn't feel like she was heard, I advised her to keep telling him. Just because someone doesn't respond the way you want them to, it doesn't mean you shouldn't tell them how you feel. It also doesn't mean you should lower your expectations. Being vulnerable doesn't mean every conversation will end the way you hope it will. Vulnerability isn't always a two-lane highway. Sometimes it is a gravel road, and the person you are meeting up with also gets caught in the dust. Modelling vulnerability with others can help them open up too, but it can take time, and practice.

If it takes too long, and there is no reciprocation, connections can be broken. Sometimes connections can be fixed, while others cannot. The thing about reaching out a hand to hold is there needs to be a willing hand on the other side to hold onto. You can stand reaching your open hand out, but if someone isn't willing to take it, eventually you will likely put down your hand.

If you find yourself in a place where you are lacking genuine connections, please be aware that there are resources that can offer a temporary one. Through many hard times in my life, I have called the Farm and Rural Stress Line. It is a toll-free mental health line we have in Manitoba. I remember crying my eyes out, more than once, to the lady on the other line. And guess what? She just listened. And listened. And when I needed to call back again, she listened some more. Sometimes we don't need someone to fix our pain. Sometimes we just need someone to be a witness to the struggle so we know what it feels like to be seen during an emotionally difficult time. It gives us permission to have those feelings and validates them, even if we have guilt about feeling them, just like the time my mom sat on my bed and cried alongside me as a depressed preteen. It is okay if something still hurts even if others don't like it or think it should. Give yourself permission to work through all feelings, whatever that looks like, and an important way to do that is getting support from wherever you can find it.

CUE UP "GIRL" BY MAREN MORRIS

There are two sayings that I often hear that really rot my ass. The first is when people say if you are going through hell, keep going. Are you kidding me? If you are going through hell, but have the ability to change something, go change it! Even if it means a different job, the end of a relationship, or some other difficult transition. Explore your options, but don't stay in hell. There is another saying that time heals all wounds. I think that's bullshit. Time doesn't heal them. We do. Time just gives us the space to process them. We have to put in the real, raw, and sometimes uncomfortable emotional work. Some people go months, years, or a lifetime without processing emotions by avoiding them. But avoidance doesn't serve our mental health. It never has and it never will. Validating emotions is the only way to honour our mental wellness.

Mental health help lines are confidential, though they may ask about the details of your situation. They offer help by listening. They may help you tell your story, determine what things you need to address, problem solve, and determine what things you have control over and what things you cannot control. If you aren't comfortable calling a mental health line, that's OK too. But what isn't OK is sitting in a difficult space alone.

Find someone you can talk to and be vulnerable with. Be real. Be raw. Talk about the hurt, even when you don't want to, and even when it makes you uncomfortable, because the weight on your shoulders will be lifted. There is no feeling in the world better than that.

It has taken a lot of time, but my husband and I are finally at a place where we can be vulnerable with each other. I can see now that he shows up for me emotionally when I need him to, and I try to do the same for him. I am also fortunate to have friends in my life who will do the same. If you don't have someone in your life who makes you feel like you have a real connection, then seek them out. It might be a new mom in a new mothers' group who might be going through the same things as you. It might be someone in your family, or even be someone you find online who you can connect with. I have a lot of female farmers who I connect with online and who can be good sounding boards. There are also a lot of public resources out there that your tax dollars are paying for. Mental health is becoming more of a priority for governments around the world. Find those resources and use them.

A good place to find connection is somewhere you probably already go every few weeks. Do you ever find yourself getting your hair cut and in some crazy deep conversation about life with your hairdresser? I'm guessing I'm not the only one who has this kind of relationship with my hairdresser. Honestly, it is great therapy to go for a haircut. You get a trim or a colour and you can sit and tell them whatever is on your mind. I don't know if they teach them in hair college how to be good listeners, or if this comes naturally to them. Perhaps it is the fact that they can't get away from you when they are doing your hair and are forced to listen. Either way, hairdressers really do play an important role in society.

Good therapy can cost a lot of money but getting your hair cut is a fraction of the price. If it is good for you to vent to someone and you just want someone who listens, then go get a trim once a month. Maybe you have someone in your life you can trust and tell anything to. That's great if you do! For others, I'm guessing that's a really rare thing. That's also where counselling can come into play. I do individual counselling and have also done couples counselling with my husband, as well as farm family counselling.

Farm family counselling might have been the most difficult but also the most rewarding counselling we have done to date! It made the structure of our farm more rewarding for everyone. James and I didn't want to raise cattle anymore because they weren't making us enough money, the time investment with a young family was huge, and my mental health was degrading without proper support at home. My sister-in-law Chery, who farms alongside us, wasn't ready to sell the cows. We were making the transition to solely grain farm and Chery did not want to make the same transition. It made for a lot of difficult conversations and compromises. I can't say enough great things about Manitoba-based Elaine Froese who coached us through that time and coaches other farm families through all the tough conversations around farm roles and farm transitions, and pretty much anything else that comes up on a farm—and there are lots! In a 2022 podcast called *Ag State of Mind* with Jason Medows, Froese speaks to the mental health crisis in agriculture. She says delaying or avoiding important conversations can erode farm family connections and sometimes erodes the farm. "This whole procrastination about not having these courageous conversations is killing agriculture and it has to stop."[66]

Counselling can also help to identify root causes of anxiety and depression. If your life doesn't allow the time or money to access counselling services, the good news is that here in Canada, some of the mental health resources are starting to get covered by provincial and federal funding. It is happening in other countries as well. Seek them out and use them. "If you think you can get through mental illness on your own, you are kidding yourself," says counsellor Erica Hildebrand. "It is imperative to find a professional who can walk you through treatment and coping skills in order to give you the best possible outcome," she says.

While I agree that professional help is best, finding support and connection, in any form, will benefit your mental health. If you are lucky enough to have someone in your life who you can be vulnerable with, share your dreams and goals, and thoughts and feelings freely, then I promise you, the connection will be very rewarding for your mental health. On the flip side of that, if you have someone in your life who you want to be more vulnerable with, take the first step. If you continually open up to someone and they don't acknowledge your feelings, honour your privacy, or they make you feel guilty for feeling a certain way, your mental health will suffer, and you either need to set a boundary with that person or find someone else to open up to.

There is a familiar saying, "Make sure everybody in your boat is rowing and not drilling holes when you're not looking." In short, make sure someone has your back, with unconditional love and good intentions, someone who will be your biggest cheerleader and help you when things get tough. If someone is drilling holes in your boat, send them overboard. The only people allowed in your boat are the ones who are going to row right alongside you. It is way easier to find people who are willing to bring you down, then to build you up. Find the former, and it will pay dividends. When you find those people, hold on tight to them. They are your cheering section. Don't ever let those people get away.

I am grateful to have friends, in addition to my husband, who will row alongside me. They hold space for me in their lives. I can text them and say, *Can you talk? I really need to talk.* Guess what? They usually do. I do the same for them. I know how important that connection is. And I value it. When one of my friends sends me a text that says, *I really need to talk,* I stop whatever I am doing, and I dial the damn phone. That's what connection is about and our mental health relies on it.

Always make sure you ask permission before you vent to someone. Make sure they are prepared and give consent before you unload on them. You can't freight train someone when they least expect it, because their reaction to whatever you have to tell them will be hard to process if they aren't prepared. The thing about connection is that it must be two-sided or it just doesn't work. You can be vulnerable all day long, but if you get nothing in return, it is time to look elsewhere. Sometimes, it takes being vulnerable with someone repeatedly, before they realize the point of connection. Not everyone will see it right away, but I guarantee that when they see and value your vulnerability, they will start to do the same with you.

Moving forward, I have made a promise that I will show up for my husband, my kids, my family, and friends as I would want them to show up for me—vulnerable, authentic, and real. Over time, I have discovered who will actually show up and be vulnerable with me, and also those who won't, and that's when I build those fences I was talking about in chapter 5. It is just that simple. I have to honour my mental health that way, otherwise it will suffer. I have also accepted that I need to continue being vulnerable with my husband going forward and trust that he is strong enough to handle whatever I throw at him (which is usually a lot). Feeling like I need to protect him from the hard stuff only makes things worse, as I've discovered in the same way I felt when my parents tried to protect me from the hard stuff. I don't want anyone to try and shield things from me and nor should I do it for anyone else.

I have learned how to hold space for my husband and he is doing the same for me. We are still really great business partners and really great parents, but we are adding "really great spouses" to the list too because we are learning how to row right alongside each other.

CUE "NEXT TO YOU, NEXT TO ME" BY SHENANDOAH

CHAPTER 11

Alcoholics and Assholes: Why It Doesn't Matter Where You Live!

Turn on your speaker and start this chapter with a song that will make you laugh.

CUE MIRANDA LAMBERT'S "FAMOUS IN A SMALL TOWN"

Let me just say that truer words have never been spoken—or sang in this case. Everyone is famous in a small town for something!

I have often received advice that the people you surround yourself with matters and that you are the product of your community. Small towns are often portrayed as places where backward thinking prevails, having a redneck is no longer a sign of long hours working in the sun, but instead an indication of how high you can jack up your truck, how many guns you own, or a way to highlight a lack of sophistication or education.

Are these misconceptions? Yes and no. I drive a truck that needs clearance because I drive across rough fields, sometimes through ditches, and every winter attempt to clear snowdrifts clogging our rural roads before the grader can clear the way. We own guns to protect our animals and our property from predators. I once had a bear eat my entire row of corn from my garden in one overnight sitting, we have lost chickens to coyotes and calves to cougars and bears, and the deer often nibble on my beets or fruit trees. I have a piece of paper on the wall of my office that I acquired after spending thousands of dollars at three different post secondary institutions. I am proud of that paper on my wall, but it holds less weight than the lived experiences on the farm. Here, education doesn't indicate your pay scale, and the geographical location of your home has no bearing on whether or not you have a small mind. (Those can exist anywhere.)

Are we a product of our community? Yes, I think that is somewhat true. But I also think it is up to us to choose what values we keep and what we need to let go. For example, small towns often have a culture of drinking. Many people drink to have fun, drink to celebrate, drink to deal with hard days, good days, drink while hunting, drink while fishing, and drink while driving a snowmobile, quad, or while driving farm equipment. Have you ever driven heavy equipment in your life? Let me tell you that when I drive equipment on our farm, my judgement never needs to be impaired. It is easy enough to make mistakes while completely sober. Sucking a stone in a combine worth a quarter or half a million dollars isn't my idea of a good time. You get the idea—a lot of small town folk use alcohol to numb emotions whether they are good or bad. I admit that it is easier to put on your whiskey glasses than to see things clearly, especially if those things hurt.

CUE UP MORGAN WALLEN'S "WHISKEY GLASSES"

I think there is a belief in many small towns that people are only allowed to publicly discuss their emotions when they are drunk enough. This can quickly turn into an addiction in people who struggle with mental health because people who experience low mood often turn to alcohol to alleviate these feelings. But alcohol, in turn, can make a low mood even lower in the long term, so this cycle is the breeding ground for addiction. Dr. Andrew Huberman is a professor of neurobiology and ophthalmology at Stanford University and has found that some people who drink regularly seem to have more cortisol released from their glands even at times when they are not drinking. Which means, your occasional few drinks might change neural circuitry in your brain as well as changing hormone circuitry by dumping additional cortisol into your body, "making people less resilient to stress, have higher levels of baseline stress, and lower mood overall."[67] People don't just get addicted to drugs and drinking; they also get addicted to escaping their reality, and these substances can be the first ticket out. Sadly, the farming and ranching world can breed these kinds of addictions. The culture of not talking or showing up for others authentically, and without alcohol, is one that unfortunately permeates more than just my small town.

I love small towns for the same reason I hate them: everyone knows your business. While they may not ask you about your business, or talk to your face about your business, they make a point of knowing your business. This can be a good thing when someone gets sick and rallies behind a family who is struggling (I just watched a small town to the south of us raise $160,000 at a community auction for a little girl with leukemia.) But I could also do without the coffee shop talk that usually takes some kind of fact and quickly turns it into fiction. That being said, I still adore small towns for the values that exist here. If I had truck trouble and was on the side of the road, not many people would drive by without asking what help I might need. If my kids are spending time in our nearby town of Angusville, they often get invited in for treats from the families who live there and are treated like one of their own. The screen doors on the porches there are very rarely locked.

There is a couple other common occurrences that happen in small towns that I find absurd and is extremely damaging to mental health. Nicknames. It seems everyone has a nickname that usually represents something you might be known for, or a mistake you made once that you might never live down thanks to the nickname you were branded with. The other thing is sarcasm. You can say almost anything and make it sound acceptable, as long as you use sarcasm and laugh afterwards. These two things degrade connection when understanding and empathy don't exist. We don't have to highlight the differences or vulnerabilities of others. Doing so degrades the mental health of those around you and simply makes you an asshole.

My guess is that if you have ever lived in a small town, you can relate to a lot of what I'm saying. Looking through a lens as someone who has struggled with mental health, I can see that even if there are some alcoholics and assholes in small towns, what I also observe is that the drinking, the sarcasm, and the lack of empathy demonstrates the wounds in our culture of not talking, the culture that has no room for vulnerability, and emphasizes poor mental health practices in a population that needs support, understanding, and connection. I know that hurt people, hurt people. With that realization, it is also the reason I would fight to help anyone and everyone who lives in a small town learn how to be authentic, vulnerable, and practice good mental health strategies like making eye contact and having conversations that will fill each other's cups, not empty them. The thing about learning a lot about mental health is that I can't get mad at people for the things they do because I usually understand everyone's reasons for doing them. I can see, through my own experiences and awareness, that there is simply a lot of mental injury in our small towns, because mental health strategies simply weren't taught here. I'm hoping to change that by modelling it for others and offering my support where needed. Writing this book is a good start. Perhaps it will spur some real conversations without requiring alcohol in the future.

You don't have to use unhealthy coping mechanisms just because people around you are. It is time to break the cycle. There is a saying that if you can't beat them, join them. It is way easier to follow this rule than go against the grain. But I'm giving you permission now: go against the grain.

CUE "SAD GIRLS DO SAD THINGS" BY PRISCILLA BLOCK

I guess you could say I have tried to play along. Sure, I have done my share of drinking and being an asshole. But I've also discovered that is not who I am. Do I want to socialize now and then and have a few drinks? Absolutely! But I don't want to navigate life that way—numbing every emotion, good or bad. I also believe I was put on this earth to use my powers for good, not evil. Therefore, I also try to control the urge to be an asshole. I think we are all aware of our own vulnerabilities, and don't need anyone to point them out for us. Those things need to be met with eye contact, an open ear, and understanding—not sarcasm.

I believe that you can live in any community and thrive, despite being surrounded by people who may have different coping strategies than you. Doing things for your own mental health shouldn't be affected by your circumstance or where you live, although if you are rurally challenged, it might just look different. Working out might mean pounding down the gravel road instead of going to a fancy gym. It might mean drinking reverse osmosis water from a well, and it might mean a bit more work to preserve vegetables from the garden so you can eat healthy all year round if you aren't close to a grocery store. It might be harder, but it is not impossible. Whatever things you prioritize in your life that make you feel good, you should be finding a way to do them despite what you have or where you live.

Do you know what else I prioritize? Practicing gratitude. I write down five things each day that I am grateful for and why I am grateful for them. This practice helps me focus on what is good in my life and has shifted my perspective for the better. Being grateful for the things in our lives can improve our mental health, and, in turn, improve our sleep, our self-esteem, and our physical health. It takes only a few minutes each day, but long term it has helped to change my perspective of how I view the world around me. I also implement this with my kids, asking them each night while I cuddle with them, "What was the best part of your day?" It is a ritual that is great for their mental health because not only are they practicing gratitude, we are also fostering connection. I highly recommend this if you have kids! It has become one of the best parts of our day.

These rituals are essential for my mental health routine, and I choose to practice them instead of conforming to what other people are doing around me. However, I think there is some truth in the saying that you are a product of your community. That's because, I know for certain, that we also have some pretty darn good values in small towns across Canada and the US. (My online farming community show me examples daily.) Don't let the title of this chapter fool you. We may be rough around the edges, but gosh we have big hearts.

You may have heard the saying, "Bloom where you are planted." I chose to bloom in Brandon when I thought I was meant to be in Nashville, and I also chose to bloom on the farm, even though I was convinced I was better off anywhere else. A good example of blooming where you are planted, is country singer Jess Moskaluke. A couple of decades ago, if you wanted to break into the country music industry, moving to Nashville seemed like the only option to land a record deal. But Moskaluke didn't move to Nashville. She garnered enough attention while remaining on the Canadian prairie to land a recording deal and build a country music career from a small town in Saskatchewan —Rocanville, to be exact, which is well known for its farmland and potash mine. Someone once told me that if you want big things to happen in small towns, you have to do them. That has stuck with me and Moskaluke is a great reminder of that.

CUE UP "MAPDOT" BY JESS MOSKALUKE

You know who else is doing big things in small towns? Truck drivers who keep our supply chain going, the people who work in construction to build our roads, the nurses and doctors in our communities, the teachers in our schools, the plumbers, electricians, and carpenters. I could go on and on. How about the florist who works out of her home in Angusville and is busy every weekend of the summer doing flowers for weddings? How about the dairy farmer from Holland, Manitoba who has a side gig taking photos of gorgeous landscapes and family pictures? The talent, determination, and resilience in small towns and rural communities is simply inspiring; but no one is immune from mental illness. I'm worried about the state of mental health in small towns and particularly in agriculture. It has been a crisis for decades where farmers and ranchers are burnt out, battling constant stressors, and aren't getting enough support when they need it.

In my farming community, there have been more suicides than I can count on one hand. In a 2020 report by Farm Management Canada called "Healthy Minds, Healthy Farms," farmers reported being less likely to get enough sleep, attend social or family gatherings, feel in control of their emotions, feel motivated about work, or seek help or advice from friends or family when under a great deal of stress.[68] Suicide is a big price to pay if the alternative is talking about how we feel, taking time for self-care, and asking for help when we need it. If talking about the hard stuff was more common and met with understanding, I wonder what change would happen in our communities. What would happen if good mental health practices were modelled for the next generation?

Poor mental health in our communities perhaps has been intensified by decades of poor economic situations, and a lack of healthy habits with nothing more to blame than the priority that most were worried only about sheer survival. First, the homesteaders who cleared this prairie of rocks and bush to make way for wheat fields, followed by those who lived through the dust bowl of the dirty 30's and the depression and, like my family, the farm crisis of the 1980's. Through all of these times, many people worried about getting food on the table and a roof over their head – those basic survival needs. Mental health was not a concept many even considered. However, that doesn't mean it didn't plague them as well. In fact, that may be the root of where this crisis was born. My husband's grandfather Charlie Melnyk, the founder of this place I call home, took his own life on our farm in 1965. It was harvest time – one of the busiest and most stressful times of the growing season. In his mid-fifties, and after spending many years working to establish his own farm alongside his wife Teenie, Charlie Melnyk shot himself on the front lawn, only after finishing morning chores. He must have known what the implications of that decision would be. He must have known that one of his family members would find him there. He must have known what kind of hurt that would cause, yet the state of mind he was in at the time must have been worse, as he felt he had no other choice. Very little is spoken here about this horrific tragedy that happened on the very soil my kids play on. Some family members have told me that they believed he was sick (with some physical ailment), and perhaps didn't want to endure suffering. My guess is whatever suffering he may have experienced or anticipated suffering, his mental health might have been the biggest ailment of all.

Anxiety and depression can cloud a person's judgment so much that reality doesn't even feel like reality anymore. Sometimes the voice inside your head can tell you such an altered version of actual events that the story you hear is very different from what others do. That's why often people will say, "I can't understand why." It is a very legitimate question, especially for outsiders looking in, who might only see a very rosy picture of someone else's life. The same can be said for agriculture, which is often portrayed as a very serene and tranquil lifestyle, while the stories of struggle seem to always be conveniently left out. The state of mind of someone who struggles with mental illness can never be fully understood by someone else, but that doesn't mean that thoughts of suicide or general mental illness can't be recognized by others. What things can others be on the lookout for?

I recently hosted a mental health course on this exact topic called "Talk. Ask. Listen." Facilitated by the Do More Agriculture Foundation, the course teaches people how to recognize someone who is struggling with mental illness or is going through a time of mental injury. Many times, those who are struggling are unwilling or unable to ask for help. They list things to watch out for such as addiction, risky behaviour, angry outbursts, and withdrawing socially.

There is hypocrisy in the agriculture industry, especially for those who raise animals on their farms. Farmers care for their animals in so many ways. They're up before dawn feeding, watering, and doctoring animals, or up throughout the night if it is calving season on a cattle ranch. Animal welfare is always a top priority. Many times, if a farmer sees an animal not interested in eating, socializing, or any sign of discomfort, then they take the steps required to make sure that animal gets what it needs. But most ranchers don't do the same for themselves or their neighbours. Charlie Melnyk was one of them, feeling the pressure to feed cows before setting out on his final chore.

Are farmer's only noble if they sacrifice themselves? At harvest time, it is a badge of honour if you combine all night. It seems to be something to brag about. One farmer will say, "We combined until 3:00 a.m. as the wind stayed up." To which another farmer will reply, "Yeah, that wind was great. Our crew went until 5:30 a.m." And while it is true that the ag industry requires long hours, I think it is important to recognize that while we can celebrate our achievements, we also need to be aware of the sacrifices that we make in the process. It is important to talk about and normalize the way we manage stress and nourish our mental wellness in the industry the same way we talk about our farming practices, our schedules, and our accomplishments.

We have to ponder questions like: Are your cows worth more than you? If your tractor or combine is low on fuel, do you bring out the slip tank and re-fuel to keep going? What happens when your own tank is empty? Do you know how to fill it back up? How often do we run on empty, sacrificing our mental health for getting a job done? I can tell you that in our industry, we have times when we can't stop working. On our grain farm, a stoppage of work can mean sacrificing thousands of dollars. If the weather doesn't cooperate with us, seeding, spraying, or harvest can mean only going to the field when the sun shines, not just when we feel mentally well. Finding time to bank sleep, when it rains or when we finish a task, taking a few minutes to stretch in the morning or walk in the evening, or reaching out to visit with a friend, might make a world of difference.

Taking the time to eat a home-cooked meal might be one of the most important things you can do on the farm to take care of your crew. If you are lucky enough to have someone to bring meals to the field, stopping for a few moments to eat a nourishing meal is the absolute best thing you can do to serve your body and mind at busy times. I would argue that the conversations over the tailgate of a truck, are almost certainly as important to feed your need for connection on those long days than the meal itself. (But gosh those meals are so good too!) My mother-in-law always makes the best meals for us and we are lucky to have her. Skip either of these things and mental health takes a hit.

Dr. James Rae, who has practiced medicine in both an urban and a rural setting in Manitoba, says he has noticed that patients in rural communities often don't get help until their mental health is at a moderate or severe stage. "I tend to see people that are at a more extreme state of distress because of a lot of the sort of cultural defaults around these things." He notes that there is a tremendous amount of stigma around mental health and trying to get help for it in a rural setting. He usually sees someone who has been struggling for a long time or struggling with intense mental health issues that verge on the side of dangerous, rather than unpleasant. "I think one of the big differences in rural versus urban practice is urban patients will tend to go see the doctor when they feel bad and rural patients tend to come see the doctor when they are not functioning."69 It often seems like an impossible task to get a farmer to go see the doctor unless they are bleeding profusely or a limb is broken, and even then, they usually won't go until chores are done. The farm seems to come first, but the farm is nothing without its farmers, and a mental injury is a wound that needs just as much attention as a broken limb.

The circumstances of farming, with constant stressors, isolation, and lack of connection is a perfect storm for mental injury. The industry has a long way to go in changing the discussions around mental health. Getting rid of the stigma, not only in agriculture but in all parts of society, needs to take top priority. We each have a choice to make mental wellness a priority, no matter what our circumstances, what industry we work in, and regardless of where we live.

CUE "SMALL TOWN SMALL" BY JASON ALDEAN

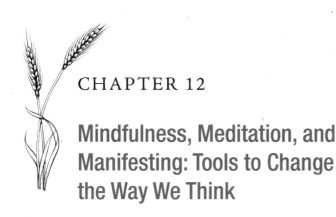

CHAPTER 12

Mindfulness, Meditation, and Manifesting: Tools to Change the Way We Think

I had a perspective change at the age of thirty-four, and it happened on a toilet. I was attending a parenting group on a Monday evening. (I can't say enough about what I learnt from a gracious soul name Dana who made me the parent I am today through her courses based in mental wellness for both parents and kids.) I couldn't stay out of the bathroom during this particular class. I kept leaving to use the washroom and it was obvious to everyone in the room that I was spending too much time in there. I thought I had the stomach flu. For the next day, I was puking and pooping and doing my best to rest. But the stomach cramping was like nothing I had ever experienced before. It was debilitating. I couldn't stand up straight and could barely walk between the bathroom and my bedroom. Toilet to bed. Bed to toilet. That was the only path I was taking. Sometimes stopping for fresh underwear because my ass was leaking. I couldn't keep clean panties on. Something was very, very wrong. This was no stomach flu. My insides were falling out. It wasn't even forty-eight hours from the onset that I crawled out of bed, near midnight, and returned to the toilet for the seventyish time that day. It was every few minutes now. I called for James because I could feel the room going black. He came into our en-suite bathroom and found me unresponsive and slumped on the toilet.

This is no knight in shining armour story like in the fairy tales. I'm getting real and vulnerable with you right now because let me tell you that real love, I-care-deeply-about-you love, the part of the vows that say better or for worse, in sickness and in health, really gets put to the test in times like this. The kind of love I am talking about is the kind when your spouse picks you up when you are passed out on the toilet, with your underwear at your feet and lays you down on a bed, trying to bring you back to consciousness. That's either love or justified fear. Maybe both. "Lewellyn, Lewellyn, can you hear me?" I could hear him, but it took me so long to be able to answer James. I was barely coherent. When I could open my eyes, I clearly saw the fear in his own. "You need to go to the hospital," he said. My body was so tired of cramping and clearly dehydrated. I knew he was right.

I assured him I could drive myself (bad judgement, I know) and told James to stay at home with the kids, who I wanted to remain sleeping. I drove myself to the nearest hospital twenty-five miles away in Russell. The drive took twice as long as it should have. I drove slow on gravel roads instead of taking the highway, scared I would pass out again, and stopping every few minutes to pull down my pants on the side of the road. In hindsight, I should have taken an ambulance but I'm not sure anyone makes good decisions when dehydrated like that. To be honest, getting an ambulance to the remote area we live always seems impossible and is a long and drawn-out affair of passing along legal land descriptions and landmarks and then waiting, and waiting some more. If an ambulance isn't in the area, one has to be brought in from another location and it can take a long time. My mom once waited an excruciating forty-five minutes for an ambulance when my son was having an asthma attack.

When I got to the hospital, the first order of business was an IV to hydrate me and a stool sample. After resisting pain meds for a few hours and waiting for the on-call lab technician to get to town, X-rays and blood work followed, though I could barely stand long enough to take the X-rays. My insides were burning with pain. My whole torso felt ripped to shreds. I couldn't stand up straight. I could only hunch over. I had been in labour with both my children for nearly twelve hours and this pain far exceeded both of those experiences. *What was wrong with me?* I wondered. I had fought through depression, I had struggled through anxiety, and now this mystery ailment was going to kill me from the inside out. *How ironic,* I thought.

CUE ALANIS MORISSETTE'S "IRONIC"

I was convinced this was going to be the end of my life. My family was visiting me in the hospital, as I lay there for days in unrelenting pain and the doctors didn't know why. I remember continually asking for morphine, one of the strongest painkillers they could give me and wondering why it didn't seem to be working that well. The stool sample results came back a few days later. It was E. coli, a bacterial infection from something I ate. After investigations, we concluded that it was probably lettuce that caused it, but I will never really know. There is no cure for E. coli, your body either fights it or it doesn't. Your fate after contracting E. coli depends solely on your physical health at the time of infection as to whether you will live to see another day or not. It took weeks for me to get back to feeling semi-normal again.

E. coli didn't kill me, but I've learned that it has been deadly for so many others. I couldn't help but think that some stupid thing I ate could have taken my life from me. After all I have been through, and the relentless fight against depression and anxiety, these circumstances were just so ridiculous. I came back from the depths of depression to have this happen?

The experience, as dumb as I thought it was, served as a kick in the ass to get my body in shape, eat healthy, and look after my physical and mental health with a renewed sense of motivation. You could say someone literally lit a fire under my ass because that's what it felt like. I can laugh about it now when I spin my lettuce in my handy Tupperware lettuce spinner, but it was life changing in the way that my perspective shifted from I'm stuck here, to now I get to be here. I wasn't going to let life happen to me. Instead, I was going to make damn sure I was living it the way I wanted. I wanted control. There's that word again. I wanted control over my health, I wanted control over my thoughts, and I wanted control over my life. My perspective changed rather quickly and my renewed motivation to be healthy had me exploring ways to better challenge my daily thoughts and explore ways to better control my mindset going forward.

Remember when I talked about Maslow's hierarchy of needs? The next few chapters are going to be touching on things that are on the top half of the pyramid. If you are struggling to meet the things on the bottom half of the pyramid, then please know these next chapters might be too much to take on at this moment and perhaps something to work on later. However, if you are at a place where you are able to do these other things, you will notice a real improvement in your mental wellness.

There are a lot of strategies that can improve cognitive restructuring. That's a fancy way of saying "changing the way you think." And that can be a really helpful tool if you deal with negative self-talk. I've heard people call them ANTs (automatic negative thoughts). We call people who have a lot of these pessimists. Simply having a bad day can make you see everything through a lens of negativity.

Even if you are an optimist, you can still have negative self-talk. Part of being self-aware is recognizing these things. You might not even know that you are doing it. The negative thoughts aren't harmful, but the feeling that you get from the thought is harmful to your mental wellness. For example, if you eat a piece of cake and think to yourself, *I really enjoyed that cake and it was delicious,* then there is no negative emotion. The emotion is that you are happy that you had a piece of cake. But if you eat a piece of cake and then immediately feel guilty that you ate it, because you don't think it served your body nutritionally or you feel guilty because you ate cake and didn't get a workout today, then eating the cake comes with a negative emotion and guilt.

I think that's also why it is important to mention that giving yourself grace with all of the recommendations I have offered is really important. In other words, I eat cake. Not every day, but you can be guaranteed that when my son or daughter spends a Saturday making a cake for the family, I will 100% of the time be enjoying a piece of it. The eighty-twenty rule is a great rule of thumb when it comes to eating well, sleeping well, or exercising—pretty much anything that you want to implement and that includes looking after your mental health. If you are doing these things 80% of the time, that is great. If you are obsessing over doing these things 100% of the time, that isn't going to help your mental health either. And chances are, you aren't going to continue doing them. You should never feel guilty about what you are doing or not doing. Always give yourself grace.

Cognitive restructuring can come in many forms. Finding a therapist is a great way to do that. But I also know that many people avoid getting professional help because of the belief that there is something "wrong" with them. Finding a good counsellor is such a great thing, but it can be hard to find one that clicks with you. It has taken me years to find one who I work well with. It can also be very expensive. We are lucky here in Manitoba: our province has been really progressive when it comes to their mental health strategies. Public funding will offer support to people who need counselling for eight to ten visits. If you live in the US, there are also county clinics that offer sliding scale fees or no fees. I think that is a great thing and anyone who needs help should be accessing these services. But if you have barriers that prevent you from getting counselling, there are so many other things you can do at home too. There are personal development authors, speakers, and life coaches who can help you change your thoughts and who can help you puzzle through a problem.

I believe we all want better mental health, but perhaps we don't understand how to achieve it. The great news is that the brain has the ability to change its physical structure as a result of learning. This is called neuroplasticity.[70] Changing the way you think takes some practice and if you haven't done it before, it can feel impossible. I can tell you from experience that it isn't as hard as you think. With practice, it has had positive effects for my own mental health. Engaging in positive self-talk, affirmations, mindfulness, meditation, and manifesting has made a huge difference in my thought processes. Just this morning, while on my third round of edits on this book which has taken about two weeks of sitting in front of my computer while also doing fundraising for the rink in Angusville, planning a fundraiser to help people in Ukraine during the war, and doing all the farm and mom things, I was feeling pretty rough. A high level of self-care is crucial during this time but even still I've had a headache for a few days now as it is all catching up to me. While I still have negative thoughts that sound like this, *Why am I even writing this book?*, I can be self-aware. I can stop them in their tracks and redirect them to reassure myself, *This isn't easy. It isn't supposed to be. But getting this book out is weighing on my heart to help others. Don't stop!* This simple affirmation to myself can keep me in the right frame of mind. James Redfield has a famous quote, "Where your attention goes, energy flows."[71] It simply means that if you focus on something that is important to you, you will work to achieve that thing. With mental health, nothing is truer. But this quote, paired with a determined soul, can sometimes degrade your self-awareness, especially when that voice in your head tells you to push through in an attempt to achieve something. It cannot be at the cost of your health.

If mental health is a goal, then perhaps our daily routines are more important than we think. Stephen Covey, author of The *7 Habits of Highly Effective People*, explains why being proactive instead of reactive is an important tool: "Reactive people are driven by feelings, by circumstances, by conditions, by their environment. Proactive people are driven by values—carefully thought about, selected and internalized values."[72]

I could list all the great quotes here and insert about one hundred pages of them, but you can find them any day of the week online or in books in your library, and you should! Knowledge is power and that is true for your mental health as well. I encourage you to always be learning. Your brain needs exercising, just like your body does, and research has shown that certain exercises can actually increase the size of the prefrontal cortex. Things like word games, learning, cooking, and math problems. My now ninety-seven-year-old grandpa works on word searches daily and his mind is sharp as a knife. I just gave you a great excuse to sit down and do math homework with your kids or grandkids. You're welcome!

Learning about why a growth mindset is more powerful than a fixed mindset has been helpful for me as well. That's because I always want to control everything. If I look at keeping an open mind and am open to other options, it usually pays off in the end. I like to call it surrendering, and sometimes that is what it feels like when you are used to controlling everything, but control, it seems, can be a killer of joy. Remember when I was talking about getting called out to the field if my husband gets stuck?

CUE "THE TRUCK GOT STUCK" BY CORB LUND

If I'm in the midst of tucking kids into bed or making supper, I might be annoyed at a change in our schedule, but going to help him get unstuck challenges my ability to emotionally regulate myself when things go sideways. Finding the ability to go with the flow and surrender control, especially on the farm, is such a great tool in order to keep myself calm and sane. The same can be said when we are in a pinch to get harvest done. Sometimes, when my combine breaks down during harvest, it can almost feel like a personal attack. (Everything is against me!) I have gotten better at being more level-headed when it comes to the emotions attached to situations like this, telling myself that my combine is tired—just like me,—it needs a bit of maintenance, and I'll get back at it as soon as we can get this fixed. I am allowed to be upset at the circumstances (validate those emotions), but regulating how I manage those emotions in a way that serves my peace of mind regardless of what the day, or weather throws at me, has been really helpful in reducing overall stress. A nasty storm can wipe out months worth of work and a year's worth of income in a matter of minutes. It is situations like this that can challenge you to your core.

My kids learned a lesson in regulating emotions when plans went awry this weekend while we were on the way to the lake to go ice fishing. It was the first ice fishing trip of the year. We packed all the things we needed for a day on Dauphin Lake: rods, bait, tent, chairs, lots of clothes, and lots of snacks. On our way there, my husband and I noticed a teenager who had slid off the highway into the ditch with his SUV. We pulled over and offered to pull him out with our truck and tow strap. But our truck's CV joint broke and our four-wheel drive wouldn't engage, and in the process of trying to pull him out, we also slid off the icy highway and into the ditch. My little boy, who was nine at the time, started a full-blown ugly cry (he gets that from his mom) and was upset that we were in the ditch, not likely to go fishing, and afraid that we will never be getting out of the ditch. I told him to breathe. I told him we had lots of clothes, and the truck was full of gas, so we would stay warm. I told him that his dad and I both had a charged cell phone, and I would call for help to get us pulled out of the ditch. I told him we had lots of food in case we got hungry. I told him the truck was safe in the ditch, and nobody would run into us because we were off the highway. I told him we also wouldn't tip because the truck was on a safe incline. I told him Mom and Dad, and his sister were all OK. We were all safe here together. And then I told him this: "It is OK to get upset. It is OK if you want to cry. But we also have to recognize what situation we are in, and how we are going to handle it."

I didn't make him feel guilty about having those feelings. I validated his fears. I talked to him about all the fear he was verbalizing through sobbing and how we settled the fear by talking over the circumstance and what we had control over and what we did not. He was scared because he didn't have control over the situation. He was scared because he wasn't sure what that meant. When we look at our fears like that, we can recognize that we can't control our fears, but we can control our emotions.

What is the difference between mindfulness and being self-aware? Not much in my opinion. Call it what you want. But I think the idea of it helps us enjoy life more when we accept the good, the bad, and the ugly. It gives space to all of those things. It allows us to accept the present moment, not because we have expectations of what it is supposed to look like, but because of what it is. It doesn't hold an expectation that the present moment will be comfortable or pleasant, because many times the real emotional rewards come from those times of vulnerability and being uncomfortable.

Sometimes too much positivity isn't helpful. Toxic positivity, as it is often called, can mask our real feelings too. We should be positive, but we also need to acknowledge and validate other emotions. While positive thinking has real benefits, I think it is important to note that while we should strive to have positive self-talk, invalidating other emotions and giving them no space doesn't fully help us to engage in mindfulness. Part of mindfulness is acknowledging all thoughts and emotions.

Mindfulness can be learned through meditation. In 2011, researchers at Harvard found that meditation can change the structure of the brain[73]—that neuroplasticity I was talking about earlier. In other words, meditation can help you stay calm in high-pressure situations. Isn't there value in that? It can also improve memory. In the last decade, scientists have discovered that every time we think, feel, or learn something new, a neural connection appears in our brain. Habits make these connections grow stronger and stronger, and over time, the connections that we don't use, grow weaker and eventually disappear. So things like worry, obsession, or negative thoughts can be trained out of our brain. (Isn't that great news for people like me?) We can train our brains by creating new neural connections, helping us to change the way we think. I find it hard to stay calm in high stress situations, but the more I practice staying calm when my combine breaks, or one of our kids get sick right before a family vacation, I know that I am building a skill so down the road I will be calmer in the future when hard stuff happens. These calmer reactions, in turn, put less stress on my body.

Do you ever look at the older generation and wonder why they seem so chill? Could it be that they are at a stage in their life where they have less stress? Maybe. Is it that they have more experience dealing with stressful situations in the past and have learnt to deal with those things in a different way? Perhaps. Stuff that you might find hard now, like trying not to freak out when one of your kids spills four litres of milk on the floor, will become easier the more and more you practice mindfulness. That's why habits are so powerful. It is literally training your brain to make something seem easy or automatic. I've started a new practice that helps me do this. Whenever something happens that is frustrating, I make sure I take a deep breath before I respond in any way. Yesterday, when my daughter and I made a batch of black bean brownies, I had two pans baking. I pulled one out of the oven and dropped it upside down, destroying every bit of brownie in the pan. I took a deep breath, a really deep one, the kind that could be heard for miles, like I was breathing out every bit of anger and rage inside of me. Then I got a pail of water and a rag and started cleaning up the mess. That deep breath helps to tell my brain, that sucked, but I can't change it, so I might as well get on with it.

Meditation does not have to be sitting with your legs crossed in a quiet room because if we are being honest, we don't all have the luxury of finding time for that. It can be as simple as concentrating on your breathing and allowing thoughts to come and go. That big breath, in tough situations, can help you make space for calming thoughts. And when you experience a negative thought, you can recognize it for just that. When you have a positive thought, you can do the same. When we recognize the way we think, it helps us to manage all our thoughts, and in turn, our emotions. Sometimes I meditate in my kitchen. And not just when I dump a pan of brownies! If you associate meditation as sitting on the floor with your legs crossed and your eyes closed, it can be that, but it can look different too. Sometimes, after my kids are home from school and have unpacked their backpacks, finished their homework, grabbed a snack, and told me 283 things about their day at school, there is a brief moment of quiet while I prepare supper. That's usually when I go into meditation mode: breathing deeply and slowly while processing my thoughts. That time of meditation follows what is usually an overwhelming time of the day for me. However, that mindful meditation, in the kitchen or wherever you are able to do it, is a great way to create new connections in the brain. Another great tip is doing guided meditations. These can be found online and many can help you through prompts to take the guess work out of how to do it. They are a great way to practice mindful meditation.

Like any other habit we develop, the more we worry, the better we become at worrying. The more we learn to stay calm and find peace, the more often we are calm and find peace. Just as exercising our brain can grow our brain, excess worry can decrease the size of our amygdala, the fear centre of our brain where those negative thoughts come from. Managing our thoughts in this way can ultimately improve our mental health.

This is also why manifesting works. Manifesting is bringing something into your life through genuinely believing it to be true. Think back to that quote from James Redfield, "Where your attention goes, energy flows." Do you remember what I wrote down on the top of my list at the personal development conference?

I wrote a best-selling book on mental health.

Affirmations are things that you either write down or see visually over and over again that you eventually believe to be true. It may not be true at the time, but you are telling your brain it is possible. I wrote that goal down for many, many weeks until I believed it to be true and achievable. Eventually, I sat down and started writing. That's why you will find goals and intentions hung on the walls around my house. You'll also find a journal beside my bed. Through telling myself that I could do it (positive self-talk), through writing down my intentions daily in a journal (affirmations), and through making a schedule that would allow time for me to write five days a week, I was able to prioritize my values and write this book. Affirmations can direct you, but don't discount the work required to get you there. Affirmations have been a great tool in my mental health journey, directing me to the things that matter the most, fill my cup, and keep me healthy.

You can manifest anything in your life. It can be a fitness goal, a financial goal, or a goal to be a better parent or better spouse. That's why controlling our thoughts can improve our life in such huge ways, because when we control our thoughts, we take ownership of the behaviours in our lives and become comfortable with both the thoughts and the actions we take, both in sync with each other. We integrate our thoughts and turn them into behaviours. In my experience, manifesting has also changed my life. It takes practice and it takes time to implement, but manifesting can be as simple as day-dreaming about the things you want in your life. Allow yourself the luxury to daydream about what you really want, then think about what tangible things can help make them a reality. I don't want to sell you on the idea that anything you want is yours. Just because you can think it, doesn't mean it will happen. It takes a lot of elbow grease to make anything happen. If you aren't familiar with that term—we use it often on the farm,—it simply means hard work. When I made my mental health a priority, I was willing to manifest what that looked like, put a plan in place, and got to work. My daily routines and habits that support my mental health don't feel like work anymore. They often feel like a privilege.

If I'm being honest, I rely more on my daily routines than my religion to guide me in my mental health journey. But I think that religion might come first for some people and that is important to note here. My past experience as a young girl, deep in depression and expected to rejoice in church Sunday morning, left me with a bit of a bitterness that lingers with me. Attending church as an adult can be extremely triggering for me. I still attend on occasion, because I know my kids have a very different experience than I had, but I still struggle with a lot of things that organized religion can teach us, mostly the idea that we should feel guilt for acting or feeling a certain way, common to Catholicism or Judaism. I don't think guilt nourishes our mental health. However, what's most important is a belief in something larger than ourselves that gives us faith and hope. If you find those things in a church, synagogue, or mosque, great! If you find that outside in nature, or with others you love, that's perfect, too! Counsellor Erica Hildebrand agrees; "My opinion is that every human being on this earth longs to find a higher purpose than themselves and that our mental, physical, and spiritual well-being is all connected and when one is off kilter, they all tend to be skewed in one way or another."

Spirituality for you might mean praying alone in your bedroom, or in a church every Sunday. Maybe your spirituality has little to no affiliation to religion. It might mean spending time in your garden or going on a long run like me. There is no right answer when it comes to spirituality. If religion is nourishing your mental health, then lean into it, but if it isn't, acknowledge that too. Spirituality can be found in many forms including and not excluding the following: religion, nature, meditation, mindfulness, manifesting, or whatever else you can find that nourishes your mental health.

CUE "LONDON RAIN" BY HEATHER NOVA

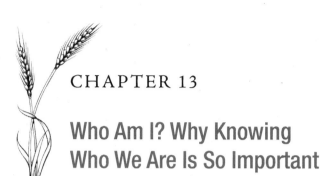

CHAPTER 13

Who Am I? Why Knowing Who We Are Is So Important

Most farmhouses are built with a porch. That's because there are so many work clothes and boots, many of them with some kind of animal shit on them. A necessity in a farmhouse porch is also a sink, so at the end of the day you can come in and scrape off the layers of dirt or grease on your hands, face, or feet before entering the home. (Who doesn't love being barefoot in the summer?) My childhood home was no different. My mom always kept an incredibly well-kept and clean home, decorating every few years with new wallpaper, or fresh paint, and with the exception of the porch, you could eat off the floor in any room at any given time. It was always immaculate, old and small, but immaculate. The porch on our 700-square-foot farmhouse had something very special attached to it. Outside our back door, was a triangular cement pad, a few inches deep that served as the Grand Ole Opry, Canadian division. The only lights to illuminate performances by my sister Brandy and I were the rays from the prairie sun, the only sound system was a cassette player we drug outside from the kitchen, and the only audience was usually a few cats and a dog. But occasionally, we used to get a visitor to the farm in a big yellow truck. Schwann's was an ice cream company that sold everything from frozen meats, pizzas, and pastries to a variety of ice cream treats. It was a home delivery service. The driver would come around every few weeks giving farm families a chance to buy some bulk frozen products. With often little to no visitors on the farm, the arrival of the Schwann's man was always a highlight. My sister Brandy and I also saw this opportunity as a time to perform our songs for an audience of one. We would belt out Reba McEntire's *"Why Haven't I Heard from You"* or Patty Loveless' *"I Try to Think About Elvis."* Cue those songs up on your headphones or speaker now or wait until later when you can perform them out loud. Trust me, they are worth the listen.

Those performances were the highlight of our summers. Music was in our blood. My great-grandfather LeRoy had started a band at the same time he was settling his own farm. My grandfather Fred and my dad Daryle both grew up playing in the band over the years, travelling to different communities to share their gift of music. The ladies in the family joined in too. I grew up with music all around me, whether it was from the stereo that sat on top of the fridge in our tiny farmhouse, the scratchy AM radio in our pickup, hymns at church, air bands with cousins, or family jam sessions in the living room at Christmas. My emotions are so tightly woven into music throughout my life, that is has become part of how I feel. It is who I am. And when in conversation with my friends and family, I often break out into song when I hear someone say a familiar lyric. That is who I am (in case the soundtrack in this book hasn't already given that away). That's also why I am at my happiest when music is playing in my house, tractor, truck or when there is any event nearby that has live music or dancing. Thankfully, we live less than two hours from the site of one of the biggest country music festivals on the prairie. Dauphin's Countryfest, the place James and I started dating, will always be one of my happy places: sunshine, camping, no work for a weekend, connection, and country music. That's my mental health medicine right there!

Music is in my bones and makes me who I am. I don't think we can truly nurture our mental health if we don't know who we are and what makes us tick. If we are trying to be more like someone else, or if we do something because we think someone else wants us to do them, we aren't living our own values. Knowing who you are, and what makes you, you, is an incredibly powerful tool.

What makes you, you? Not mom you. Not wife you. Just you. Maybe you have been living so long trying to please or raise others that you don't even know what things you value anymore. Or maybe you just haven't made the time to think about what you value. If you haven't, now is the time.

Psychologist Dr. Jenn Hardy writes on another one of her Post-it notes, "It's hard to tune into your intuitive voice if you never let yourself slow down enough to actually hear it."[74] I think for some, but not others, the COVID lockdowns really slowed life down enough that people found something out about themselves in the solitude. What they found was that they either really liked the way they were living their life or that their current way of living wasn't serving their mental health because it wasn't in alignment with their own values, but instead was in alignment with what they thought were their values, either learned from family or society. COVID made space for people to re-evaluate their values in such a great way.

My values list looks like this:

- Music and dancing
- Alone time (because I am a highly sensitive person and need to recharge)
- Family time
- Connection with others who show unconditional love
- Time with nature
- A passion for learning and health
- A desire to help others

What does that look like in my life? This is how I translate those values into my life through actions and what they look like:

- Running, gardening, listening to music, and dancing
- Making healthy meals
- Cuddling with my kids every night before bed
- The beach, the sound of loons on a summer night, and campfires with my family
- Reading, writing, and taking pictures
- Singing—any chance at karaoke and I'm taking the mic!
- Hanging out with good friends
- Country music festivals and concerts
- Driving my Honda side by side or my pickup down gravel roads in the warm summer air
- Travelling and new experiences
- Achieving goals at a pace where I can show up in a meaningful way for myself, my husband, my kids, and my friends
- Living and working on the farm

CUE "IN MY VEINS" BY LAUREN ALAINA

If you haven't already, make your own list. Make one of your values. Now make one of the actions you do that represent those values. How do they translate into your behaviours and your actions? If you value your health, are the actions you are taking nourishing your health? If you value family, are you really showing up for your family in the way you want to?

Taking care of your mental health is an investment of time, in the best future possible. If you are going to feel healthy and happy, there is one thing are you going to need along the way that can really throw a wrench in your plans if you don't have it: confidence. When you have it, the world is a better place. You can't just wake up one day and say, "I am going to have confidence." To be clear, having confidence does not equal being an asshole. Let me write that again: *Confidence DOES NOT give you permission to be an ASSHOLE.* Confidence doesn't mean that you always have to be right, or know it all, and it definitely doesn't mean that you push your beliefs on others. I think some people believe that confidence is belittling other people or putting them down to build yourself up. Nope, again, that's called being an asshole.

Confidence, in my opinion, should mean trusting yourself, trusting your thoughts and feelings, and not giving them a label as right or wrong, and not pushing them on others, but making others aware of what you think and feel without judgement. You should be able to share your thoughts or feelings freely while being considerate of others, knowing that they may not share the same beliefs.

CUE "CONFIDENT" BY DEMI LOVATO

You can be confident and still be kind. There is a word for this: respect. We don't always have to agree with one another, but we do have to respect one another. Looking out for your own mental health also means looking out for the mental wellness of others around you. Dr. Jody Carrington is a psychologist who gives advice about mental health. She has written a number of books on the subject, speaks to audiences across the country and online. One of the most important things she teaches is that the mental health of children can only be as good as the caregivers around them (parents and teachers are the foot soldiers for mental health in kids). Her message is one that looks at how mental health strategies in our communities and schools can only be improved when we work together, and I love her message about tackling mental health issues, often telling her audiences that we were never meant to do this alone. *This* meaning the hard stuff. *This* meaning the good stuff. *This* meaning life. Another piece of advice she often offers up to her audience is this: "Be kind and don't tolerate bullshit. In that order." I can't think of any better advice.

Building confidence in your ability to manage your own mental health is kind of like being in a new relationship with someone and building trust. At first, you don't know if they are going to break your heart, but as time goes on, you build trust. When you move in together or get married to someone, you might have to share a chequing account or financial obligations. That would also require trust.

When James and I got married and our big Ukrainian-style wedding was over, we took count of all the money we received for gifts from family and friends. I suggested that we pay whatever bills were left owing from the wedding, and the rest should be put in a savings account earmarked for building a new home as we were still living in a house trailer. My husband suggested that we take the money and invest it into the farm. Reluctantly, and after much discussion, I agreed, knowing that the farm needed cash flow, and I trusted that we would see return on that investment. Five years later, we would start construction on a new home. It would take two years to build, but after a large investment of time and money, we moved into our new home in 2015 and said goodbye to our drafty and sometimes mouse-infested house trailer that had a tendency to freeze water and sewer pipes during the winter months. I trusted that our investment in the farm would be the right decision, and in the end, the return was more than that savings account would have produced.

Building trust in a relationship can be much the same as building confidence in yourself. It takes time, and you have to trust that the decisions that you make and the way you live your life, is the best for you, and only you. We make thousands of decisions each day, some are as small as what you are going to wear or what radio station you will listen to in the car, but others are more important to our physical and mental health like what you are going to eat, how and what kind of exercise you will get, how much time you will spend on work in a day, how much time you will spend with family in a day, or what you are going to read?

Can you get burned even as you have confidence in the moment and trust in the situation? Absolutely! Trust isn't something that always ends well. It most often reveals itself over time.

The Oxford English Dictionary defines trust as the "firm belief in the reliability, truth, or ability of someone or something."[75]

Could the farm have had a few bad years, and could we have lost our wedding money and been unable to build a new home? Absolutely! But the thing with trust is, you never actually know the outcome. You surrender control. You can only know the process and understand the risk. You have to be comfortable with the unknown and be willing to be uncomfortable sometimes. Gosh, if that doesn't describe farming, I don't what does.

In life, you can only ever control your attitude and your effort. I hate using this phrase because it is so overused, but it really is just putting it in plain and simple terms. You can control what you put in your mouth. Will it be carrots or French fries? You can control whether or not you are going to go for a walk or a run before you go to work, you can control what time you go to bed at night to ensure you get enough sleep, and you can damn well control how you treat yourself and treat others. When you trust in yourself, that you will make those decisions with only the best intentions, then you can truly have confidence. And when you make a decision that you internalize as being a bad decision, don't beat yourself up. Own that you made that decision. Did it serve you? Or did it not serve you? Could you make a different decision next time that might serve you better? Analyze your decision making, and over time, that trust gets better in yourself. Prove to yourself that you can rely on your decision making. Does changing your belief system or your opinions over time make you a hypocrite? Absolutely not! You are always free to change your mind, as you learn and grow and discover new things, and it absolutely does not make you a hypocrite—it just makes you wiser. The important thing to remember is to always believe, wholeheartedly, that the only person who can make the right decision for you is you! Have you heard the saying, "You do you?" Without a doubt, no one is more qualified to make decisions for you. Trust your intuitive voice.

If you are reading this and that voice in the back of your mind says, *I can't trust myself,* I'm here to tell you that you can. Maybe that means reading more books, finding new recipes to cook in order to eat healthier, finding a workout program to get more exercise, setting an alarm on your phone to tell yourself to go to sleep at a certain time or get up a certain time, or maybe it simply means listening to your gut about what feels right. Maybe it means making an appointment with a therapist to deal with some really heavy crap that you haven't dealt with in your life. Maybe it means having some real, raw, and honest conversations with some people in your life. Be honest about what you need. Only you know what that is. I've done them all. While some benefited me more than others, books really fed an appetite for knowledge and that knowledge kept giving me more confidence. I love reading books about how I can be better, do better, live better. I love to learn. Because I am an Enneagram One, it also means I hold self-improvement as a value and am always motivated to learn something new, in particular, learning about psychology. It means I am a voracious reader and a lifelong learner.

When my kids were small, I didn't take the time to read. I just didn't have it. I was at the bottom of Maslow's hierarchy of needs and with two small kids I was living in survival mode. However, as my kids got older, I took up reading again. I wanted to pick a book about health, because, as you can probably guess by now, that topic of health and self-improvement intrigues me and of course, I was dealing with anxiety and didn't know where to turn. My newly discovered love for running as a tool to manage my anxiety led me on a book search regarding the topic of health. I searched the Internet for reviews on good books about the topic. I found a book called, *What Makes Olga Run? The Mystery of the 90-Something Track Star and What She Can Teach Us About Living Longer, Happier Lives*. In the book, author Bruce Grierson tells the story of a ninety-three-year-old track star. He researches how our bodies and minds age. He explores what factors influence health and longevity.[76]

The first book I read in years set me on a journey for living better and started building my confidence. It was so inspiring that I made a commitment to myself to always stay active. The science had convinced me that if I started now in my thirties, I could almost certainly replicate the trail that Olga blazed making centenarians an age group that could certainly be as active as I was now. I thought, if running was providing so many benefits to my life now, what could I do over the next fifty, sixty, or even seventy years? It was so inspiring that I passed the book along to my grandfather (who replicated a lot of Olga's traits and is perhaps why he just celebrated his ninety-seventh birthday), my step-grandma, who then passed it on to my mom and dad. I wanted all the aging people in my life to know her story and I wanted to shout it from the mountain top: *keep moving people!* If we keep moving now, the tangible benefits will show up when we are ninety-seven and are still able to get up off the toilet by ourselves.

The book was a good start to my personal development journey. It built confidence in my mental health journey too. From there, I explored other books about exercise, diet, marriage, and many books about mental health. I discovered that there were so many authors who were researching and sharing their experiences. I was learning through my own journey and others as well. The more I read, the more confidence I had. I was armed with knowledge and was always determined to embrace a growth mindset and try whatever new things I was learning. I learned what was best for me and what wasn't.

One author whose authenticity really brought out the best in me was Rachel Hollis. She taught me, along with many other women, to be unapologetically myself and not to make myself smaller around other people. Her words and encouragement helped me to understand my worth. "Be the kind of woman who never asks permission to be herself," she preaches in her book, *Girl, Stop Apologizing.*[77]

Simply put, that is the key to confidence. Have enough tenacity to believe, without a doubt, in the value you bring to the world. The other lesson that she preaches (I say preaches because she is an amazing communicator and is a preacher's daughter) from her book *Girl, Wash Your Face* is that, "Someone else's opinion of me is none of my business." This quote is adapted from the title of another self-help book by Terry Cole-Whittaker, *What You Think of Me Is None of My Business.* In short, this is some of the best advice for small-town living. People will always have something to say about everything or anything you do, so if it makes you happy, you might as well do it anyways! You do you. We aren't all the same and we were never meant to be. Hollis adds, "Comparison is the death of joy, and the only person you need to be better than is the one you were yesterday." This is so true for females working in the agriculture industry. Females in the industry often get ridiculed for not being dedicated enough (because God forbid we prioritize raising little humans), not being strong enough do some of the heavy lifting, and this one gets me every time—too pretty to be a farmer. I read a thread on Twitter recently that made fun of a female farmer because she had her hair and makeup done and posted a selfie on her farm. The flood of comments about how much she does in a day or the legitimacy about her being a farmer was absolutely disgusting. As soon as a confident woman has something to say (or a picture to post) in the industry, someone will surely have something to say about it. I'm over it. That's because women outnumber men on our farm. Without the women on this farm, it wouldn't be what it is today and I often credit Baba Teenie Melnyk for what she endured after Charlie's passing. The same can be said for the men here too. We have all made an incredible investment of time and effort, and it isn't a competition between genders. We are a team that works together with different roles, but with the same goal. Some days I may be dirty in my coveralls and boots with my hair a mess, or I might have my hair and makeup done. My appearance, I can assure you, does not dictate my role on this farm or my value as a farmer.

Whether you are a farmer or simply work in the industry, there is this comparison that exists between males and females that drives me bonkers. Some people might think that I am a firm believer in gender equality, and I'm the first to confess I will advocate for women always, but if you want complete disclosure, my physical ability is far more limiting on the farm than the fact that I have a vagina. My husband can lift heavy shit. My body composition simply cannot compare to his no matter how many weights I lift. However, while I think gender should never inhibit you from trying or doing something, I have come to realize that finding the right role for you, regardless of your gender, is far more important. I don't let the things I struggle to do become insecurities. I learn as I go, and focus on what I'm good at – thing like doing the farm books, and budgeting. I am a careful equipment operator and a good decision-maker, but when it comes to pulling wrenches, I don't have the strength or know-how that my husband has. I have a female farmer friend who does not want to drive equipment, but she rocks field meals like no one I've ever met. I operate equipment on our farm, but neither is right or wrong and we don't need to compete against each other whether we are male or female. Finding your role, in life or work, that suits you and the situation you are in, should be your only goal. For example, my husband and I can both back up a trailer. Has he done it a few hundred times more than I have? Sure. Can I do it as well? Sure. While we can do some of the same things, we depend on each other for others knowing that we don't have to do it all. We each have skills in different areas, and it isn't a competition. We are on the same team. I'll gladly let him back up a set of Super B grain trailers knowing that he is the better semi driver in this relationship, while he'll leave the farm books to me. Recognizing our strengths, supporting each other in those roles, no matter what they are, is far more important than competing.

Some Twitter followers haven't fully understood this notion yet. So, I'm here to tell you: what we do does not determine our worth as a person, but having confidence will help us to be who we are, free of opinions and comparisons from others. Having confidence means, "I won't break myself down into bite size pieces to serve others. I will stay whole and let them choke." That anonymous quote says it perfectly. My opinion is that I will be exactly who I am, wear whatever I dang well please, and celebrate every single dang win along the way.

My mental health and honouring who I am as a highly emotional being will always take priority over other people's opinions because I have the confidence to know that being me, simply me, is the best medicine for my mental health. The power in that one realization has been huge. That doesn't mean I don't consider the opinion of anyone (I'm not an asshole). It just means prioritizing mine, and the ones who live under the same roof, and beyond that, the rest are taken with careful consideration: Do they provide unconditional love? Are they honest with me? Do they fully understand the situation before having an opinion? If we stop caring what other people think, connection can be lost, but if we care too much, we lose the ability to be vulnerable. Consider other people's opinions carefully and remember yours matters the most.

Knowing who we are is so important. What makes you tick? What fires you up? Self-reflection and self-awareness are key components to confidence, self love, and good mental health, because you can't love someone you don't know. This next song perfectly explains why you should never doubt yourself. If anyone should have your back, it should be you.

CUE UP "DOUBT ME NOW" BY CODY JOHNSON

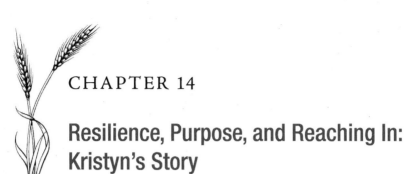

CHAPTER 14

Resilience, Purpose, and Reaching In: Kristyn's Story

Circumstances can change your life, but so can goal setting with a side of grace.

CUE SAWYER BROWN'S "THE RACE IS ON"

In the fall of 2020 during harvest, the busiest and most rewarding time of the year, we combined for a total of seventeen out of twenty days during the month of September to get over 3000 acres of crop in the bin. We didn't mess around, we had good weather, and we took full advantage of it. That's because there were invisible scars from the two years previous. In both 2018 and 2019, we struggled for well over fifty days through rain, sleet, and snow to get the crop harvested. Getting the grain in the bin meant that we could make our payments, pay our bills, and continue to grow the farm.

During those difficult years when weather wasn't on our side, and we finally rolled the combines back into the shed at the end of harvest as the snowflakes were flying, it felt as though we had accomplished the unthinkable. At times, it seemed a lot of our crop might stay out all winter under the snow. The fear of not being able to make our payments is always a very real concern, but in 2018 and 2019 it was very palpable. In the end, we were able to get the crop off, but not without a lot of adversity, in less-than-ideal conditions.

In contrast, 2020's harvest felt like a breeze. That didn't make it any less important. Sometimes the journey to a goal is smooth sailing, and sometimes it kicks and screams. But determination is built into the adversity of the journey.

When things get tough here on the farm and it snowed on our crop and our combines, we didn't go park the combines for the year. We were frustrated, no doubt. But we waited until the sun came out to dry the crop enough to try again.

And when it snowed a second time, we waited it out again. And when we had to combine around snow drifts, we did that too. And when we had to dry grain from harvest time until Christmas, we did that too! Does it suck? Absolutely! Is it hard? For sure! Did it add a few wrinkles to our faces and some grey hairs to our heads. Sure did. But it also built grit and resilience. It also made us grateful for the journey this year when Mother Nature was a little easier on us.

These kind of stressors in farming are no different than any tough time you might experience throughout your life because of circumstances out of your control. My husband and I lived in survival mode for weeks when we had doubts about the harvest. It was a good example of how circumstances out of our control can be the biggest threats to our mental health. But we have to look at the potential for growth during times of adversity. These are the times that have the most potential to build strong mental health practices. I've learnt that happiness does not mean we have no problems. We will always be presented with challenges throughout our life. Happiness means we have the capacity to deal with those problems or challenges as they come.

Trauma is also something that, if not matched with good mental wellness practices, can leave a lifetime of mental injury. Kristyn Eftoda has lived through unimaginable heartache. The kind of heartache that can leave someone mentally injured for a lifetime if they aren't intentional about validating and honouring their emotions. But her story is one of resilience, and I think it is an important example to share. She has used many of the techniques in this book to counter the mental injury when her world was turned upside down. She credits the support from her community for reaching in when she couldn't reach out.

Kristyn and Wade Eftoda met in high school in Roblin, Manitoba. Kristyn was fifteen, and Wade, sixteen. He already had his licence, and the tall, dark farm boy would cruise around after school most days in his 5L red Ford Mustang. After the two connected at a high school party, Wade made sure to keep his eye on the cute, little blonde firecracker. Most days, he would leave school just in time to catch Kristyn walking on the sidewalk and would often offer her a ride to work. This little ritual went on for weeks, the conversation was easy and a friendship formed that Kristyn describes as feeling, "exhilarating, reliable, and easy all at once."[78] After a few weeks of this, Kristyn leaned in during the after-school drop off one day and said, "I don't know if you know this or not, but I like you and I'm just curious when are you going to ask me on a proper date?" Surprised, but relieved, Wade agreed and many dates followed, and so did a wedding in 2009. The high school sweethearts grew to be best friends, never spent much time apart, and shared such great love that their connection was evident to anyone who knew them.

Kristyn was an elementary school teacher in Inglis, Manitoba and Wade worked at a local seed and chemical retailer there as well. They had plans to farm alongside Wade's family and had decided to build their forever home on his parents' farm with Wade doing much of the work himself with the help of family and friends. They moved in during the fall of 2016 with a toddler in tow. Three years later, they were learning to manage life as a busy family of five that included six-year-old son, Liam; three-year-old daughter, Evony; and a newborn, a son named Boyd.

On March 3, 2019, only six weeks after Boyd was born, everything changed. Wade had gone on a snowmobile derby, an annual fundraiser for the Inglis Fire Department. The derby welcomes people from the community and the surrounding area to come for a ride on their snowmobiles on a marked trail, offering a chance at prizes and of course a homemade warm meal when people return put on by community volunteers. The event was a big deal in Inglis, and Wade wasn't about to miss it, especially when he was given a chance for his first day of fun with friends and family since he and Kristyn became a family of five with three kids under the age of six.

It was cold that day. Windchill factors were hitting minus forty. But the cold weather didn't deter most riders, including Wade who rode the nearly forty miles of trail to the Shell Valley and back to town. Wade returned to the Inglis hall, which was the start and finish line for the derby, and sat down to have a warm meal and visit with friends before heading home on his snowmobile alongside his dad and a couple of friends.

Kristyn remembers thinking that night that it was odd that he wasn't answering his phone when he didn't return at the time she expected him to, but she assumed he was visiting with friends a bit longer or was out of cell service, something very common in rural communities. Worried about him and waiting for his return, she knew something was wrong the instant her parents, alongside Wade's mom, drove up to the house just after midnight. She watched Wade's mom Rose get out of the car first and says she will never forget the look in her dad's eyes when he told her that Wade was gone. Wade had suffered an accident while on his way home from the derby. He hit a tree with his snowmobile and died instantly. Kristyn's dad, Claire, caught her as she fell to the floor and held her tight. "If it weren't for them blocking the door, who knows what I would have done. I just kept saying 'No, no, no, I can't live without him.'" In the days that followed, Kristyn explains that she felt like she was living outside of her body. "I was a completely empty shell," she said.

CUE "DROWNING" BY CHRIS YOUNG

The heartbreak was unlike anything Kristyn had ever experienced. "I had lived a pretty charmed life up until Wade died," she admits. But so much had changed after his death, including her mental health. "I have a lot of amnesia a few months before and after Wade died, but I can tell you that I can count on more than one hand how many times I said, 'I hate my life.' I realize now that I was feeling something, but I was only living in a three-dimensional world that seemed flat at times. I didn't hate my life, but I wasn't practicing gratitude, building resilience, reflecting, growing, and loving to my full potential."

Something sparked a change in Kristyn. She didn't want to live in a pity party she could have made for herself. Rather, at a time of unimaginable grief and loss, Kristyn set out on a mission for something to keep her going, and she realized she had three of them, all of whom resembled their father who she loved so much. She started reading books about grief and answering her kid's questions about death. "Some of the questions made my stomach turn," she says, but answering them honestly helped her and her kids have a healthy relationship with grief and death, always highlighting their dad's love for them.

"My mental health at the time was pretty much incomprehensible," she recalls of the time following Wade's death. She was struggling with survivor guilt, feeling at times that Wade would have been the better parent. "I remember telling a friend of mine that I have never felt depression and that was my biggest fear, next to never seeing my husband again." Determined not to go into "the dark" as she refers to mental illness, she focused on staying in survival mode for months following the accident. "I knew that if I didn't set a goal or a dream for myself, I would succumb to just living to pass by the days." At first, breastfeeding Boyd became her purpose, as she had a newborn who needed her. Putting her own needs to the side at first, her kids became her purpose for living. She said looking after herself and loving herself came later. She credits the community for reaching in when she couldn't reach out for helping that transition to happen.

The help from friends, family, and her small-town community started pouring in. Kristyn discovered there was a new freezer full of meals in her garage, a fund-raising campaign had been started for her and her kids, and she says just minutes after hearing of Wade's death, friends were in her kitchen sweeping the floor and offering help with the house and the kids wherever she needed it. "I can't stress the community support enough…it made me feel less alone…I know it is essential to stay connected." Kristyn adds that, "Grief is a deeply personal thing and each person grieves in a different way." She was happy that people reached out but noted that others might have needed more space, recognizing this in the different reactions she saw in her family and friends who were also grieving. "Let the griever take the driver's seat but don't be afraid to sit in the passenger seat with them."

Kristyn contacted a therapist who gave her a prescription on her first day—sleep! A month later, she added yoga to help get a hold of her anxiety and manage the fears she was now facing. One of her biggest fears was raising three kids as a solo parent. "Wade was the kind of man who would do anything to keep you safe. Without him, I was going to have to not only keep myself safe, but my kids, too."

During the first year following Wade's death, Kristyn started getting anony-mous gifts and messages from people in the community. A group of ten women, who called themselves the Secret Sisters, each took on one month and dedicated their time to reaching in to Kristyn and her kids when they needed it most. They sent cards with balloons or stickers, planned activities for her and the kids, planned a night at a restaurant or a day at the salon. "The Secret Sisters, I'm sure, saved my life," Kristyn says about the experience. Adding that while she benefited from their efforts, the kids did too. "It gave them a little bit of magic and it gave them a little bit of fun and all the ideas and adventures kept me going on the right path."

With the help of family and the Secret Sisters, Kristyn was prioritizing sleep, exercise, nutrition, mindfulness, and connection, and her mental health was taking a turn for the better. "It was so important for me to be reminded of healthy eating and exercise. I didn't have the cognitive ability from the exhaustion of grief to see those things as unselfish and necessary acts of love," she says.

She adds, "I cannot say exactly when it happened, but with therapy, a supportive village, and my three little lights, a version of myself emerged, determined to use my new perspective to honour my husband and live my life for the two of us. I have always been a driven, hard-working person with a desire to fix things. In the beginning, I was determined to fix my grief, but I have learned that this cannot be fixed, only experienced."

Kristyn says validating all the emotions of grief makes way for resilience. She found validation in books, some that were written by other widows. "I vigorously read books to build my compassion, mindfulness, and connection skills. I dug into the ashes to find my grit, motivation, and courage, and become a present, active member of my life again striving for resiliency, gratitude, and self-love," she says. Kristyn knew she was accepting her circumstances and validating her emotions when she started using sentences that started with "My husband died…" After a few weeks, Kristyn says a new perspective emerged. "I was seeing the smallest things so clearly, feeling intensely connected to nature and others, and noticing how things felt in my body." Adding that she was "relearning how to function."

Kristyn believes that to honour our mental wellness means that we need to "turn towards the hard stuff. And once we do that, our bodies can heal from the trauma and we can feel joy again." She says sometimes, "Joy and pain must coexist so we can move forward with grace."

Validating the emotions that the kids and her feel at every stage is the only way to honour their mental health. She says, "It's not unhealthy to keep his life and memories very much alive. He can and will always be a part of our story. His book may have been closed, but ours didn't and we will continue to write him in. It is the only way for our kids." Validation, at every stage, has helped them to move forward.

Eye Movement Desensitization and Reprocessing (EMDR) therapy helps people recover from trauma and other distressing life experiences, including PTSD, anxiety, depression, and panic disorders. It is designed to resolve unprocessed traumatic memories in the brain. Kristyn says EMDR therapy helped her to file away some memories and feel more compassion for herself. "I have realized through EMDR and regular therapy that I can't control what has happened, but I have some control over my thoughts about what has happened," she says. "I have learned that I can try to carry [my kids'] grief backpacks with mine and bear that heavy load for them, but there is no point really. They must carry their own, whether empty or full, because they will grieve slowly for the rest of their lives and so will I in a different way. I'm better off just carrying my own so that when theirs gets really heavy during the big moments I can let them lean on me and I will be stronger and ready to guide them." She adds, "Being a mother has proven to be the most challenging, rewarding, and important role I will ever have."

She is finding purpose in other ways too, deciding to apply for her master's in education in 2020 with a goal of teaching others how to process grief. "Ever since taking my kids to play therapy, I had been fascinated with child psychology." She decided that going back to school was the right choice has focused on a new goal: teaching grief in the classroom. Part of her master's included writing narrative inquiry as well as sharing her story with others. "Writing has become my creative expression," she says. Adding that the courses have challenged her to "think more about grief and how we treat it in the school and classroom, and it has given me a productive, safe place to process my grief." She says going back to school has brought her so much joy and wonders if counselling in schools might be the best way to make meaning out of her loss. "I have become interested in brain science, emotional intelligence, and types of therapy that rewire our thoughts," she says.

Kristyn refers to four books that got her through some of the toughest moments following Wade's death: *It's OK That You're Not OK* by Megan Devine, *Healthy Healing* by Michelle Steinke-Baumgard, *Just One Thing* by Rick Hanson, and *Resilient: How to Grow an Unshakable Core of Calm, Strength, and Happiness* by Rick Hanson. She says these books opened herself up to being vulnerable with people and recognizing the value of self-acceptance. She says everyone could benefit from a better understanding of grief and how it affects our mental health. Referring to Megan Devine's work, she says, "It addresses the issue that grief is scary and our culture tries to avoid it even though life and death are the only two guarantees on earth." Kristyn says it always made her feel worse when people would see her and say nothing or just pretend she didn't exist. "I see them, they look away, head down, like I'm a ghost." She says compassion and understanding of grief is one way to nourish our mental wellness. Adding that even a comment like, "Nice pj's, glad to see you out and about," from someone in the community would offer the validation she required to accept the transition to healing. She also notes that hearing other people's stories about Wade has been healthy for her mental health, and says avoiding those conversations don't honour his life or the mental health of the living. So next time you find yourself with someone who is grieving, remember this: sometimes the best thing you can do with someone who is grieving is not to stay strong, but instead, crumble alongside them. Healing can happen in the hurt.

While Kristyn has used a variety of resources to improve her mental health, COVID added another element of anxiety. Reluctant to take medications in the past, in 2020 Kristyn started taking some medication to manage her anxiety, as well as some vitamins and supplements that she says have made an improvement in her overall mood and mental health.

Kristyn credits the resilience she has learned in grief that has put her on a new path, living forward, with purpose: "[Wade] lived and loved as if each day was his last." He would tell Kristyn before his death that, "only you can create your own happiness." The messages he left with her, along with her passion for teaching, her three little lights, and her master's in guidance and counselling are her life goals now. "I wake up each morning saying 'Good morning, I love you' to myself and go to bed each night saying, 'Goodnight, I love you' to my husband. This is my constant reminder to love myself as hard as he loved me."

Kristyn is proof that mental wellness can be achieved under any circumstance, and especially within times of adversity, as long as you are committed to making mental wellness a priority. Her story also emphasizes the important role of our communities.

CUE UP "THE CLIMB" BY MILEY CYRUS

There is a popular saying: "Falling down is part of life. Getting back up is living." That is the most basic way of explaining adversity in any journey and the resilience that can come out of it. Does falling down mean that we can't lie on the floor for a little while and have a pity party? Nope. We are allowed to do that. In fact, I encourage you to do that. Have yourself a big ole pity party with balloons and cake if you want! Or stay in bed for the whole day. You are allowed to feel unpleasant emotions. In fact, you need to feel them. We have to learn to validate emotions and give them space. It is the only way to honour our mental health. We can't heal it, if we don't feel it. If we ignore the things that hurt, their effects can linger for years, or even a lifetime. That's why I encourage you to feel all the yucky emotions, talk about the tough stuff and take the time to heal the things that hurt. Whenever your pity party is over, you will get back up even stronger. Like a seed needs moist, warm soil to germinate, resilience is only found after adversity is met with vulnerability.

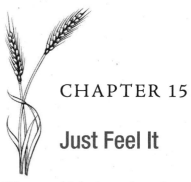

CHAPTER 15

Just Feel It

Winter and I don't get along. Let me rephrase that: I f*cking hate winter. I hate the cold, and it hates me. I dread every bit of Manitoba winters. I hate unthawing waterers in the dead of winter with frozen fingers, shoveling and trudging through snow, and days that have very few hours of sunlight- the kind of days that can allow the darkness to seep inside my soul. When the summer starts to fade and the autumn leaves burn red and orange, I get this feeling that the trees are bleeding out all the beauty they can muster before winter arrives. It always makes me stop and stare, take a deep breath, and gives me chills before the actual big chill arrives with loads of snow and bitter cold. I try to savor that change in the season. In the blink of an eye, the trees lose their leaves as fast as they changed colour, and nature suddenly seems cold, lifeless, brutal, and barren. I know it isn't permanent, and I know in a few months new life will begin again, but feeling stuck in that lifeless environment for four to five months continues to make me uncomfortable year after year of living here. But we aren't meant to be comfortable all the time. Comfort isn't what makes me thankful when I see the first green sprouts in the spring. Winter is a rest period for nature. It can't sprout new growth and bloom gorgeous colours without having a rest. I have learnt that embracing the uncomfortable winters as a rest period for myself can be life-giving and has also served as a good reminder to be grateful for the busy, beautiful, and fulfilling times on the farm. Even in the stressful or overwhelming times, I'm usually hit with a breathtaking sunset while straight cutting a field of wheat, or I find myself face-to-face with my giggling kids in the garden while picking armfuls of produce.

As a young girl growing up on the farm, I would resent the workload that came with farming, feeling that it pulled me and everyone away from what I valued most: connection. I can tell you that feeling hasn't gone away. In fact, I think that might be the toughest thing about farming. It is a challenge to fit those connections into every day. We sacrifice so much to have this profession, but connection cannot be one of them. While this profession is full of challenges and so many things we cannot control, it bursts with beauty through the seasons, and provides the most basic connection of all: our connection to the land. It is that connection that has kept me rooted in this place. The screams of thunder from wicked summer storms and the charm of a calm sunny day are akin to the experiences that come with cultivating the dirt and the life we live here.

I always read about mental illness and wondered why life experiences never seemed to play much into diagnosis until I read a study from the University of Liverpool that concluded psychiatric diagnoses are scientifically worthless as tools to identify mental health disorders.[79] One of the key findings of the research was that "almost all diagnoses mask the role of trauma and adverse events." Another finding pointed out that "diagnoses tell us little about the patient and what treatment they need." Lead researcher Dr. Kate Allsopp called the diagnostic labels such as schizophrenia, bipolar disorder, depressive disorders, anxiety disorders, and trauma-related disorders, "scientifically meaningless."[80] If that is the case, people who experience neglect, abuse, trauma, or loss may be left to slip through the cracks when seeking meaningful mental health support. It also leaves me thinking that perhaps the rural population is dealt one of the hardest hands when it comes to adverse life experiences. They may be known as the most resilient and the toughest group, but at what cost? While vulnerability and authenticity may be required within rural communities, they may also need empathy and understanding from the paved streets that rely on them, from the governments that regulate them, and from the institutions that surround them.

Currently, our farm is facing inflated land costs as we compete with investors for farmland and are also watching interest rates and input costs rise. Farmland is becoming increasingly difficult to acquire for family farms like ours, or anyone who wants to enter the industry. Despite the struggles, there is an immense sense of pride that comes from working the land. Farm families dedicate their lives to produce fuel, fibre, and feed for livestock, and food for consumption around the world. Throwing on a pair of work boots and producing these things while being stewards of the land is a task only a few will experience, and that number keeps getting smaller. In 1925, 30% of the population were farmers in North America. According to Statistics Canada, less than 2% of the population feed nearly thirty-seven million people in our country today.[81] In the United States, only 1.4% of people work in the agricultural sector according to the USDA, feeding 330 million people in that country, and many commodities are exported on both sides of the border to feed people around the world.[82] The global population is expected to increase by 2.2 billion by 2050, which means farmers will have to grow about 70% more food than what is now being produced, according to the American Farm Bureau.[83] It makes me wonder if consumers know the sacrifice happening on farms so they can buy their food at the grocery store. Or as The Reklaws sing in their song "Where I'm From," do they, "think it's all backroads, bonfires, cornfields, and country music?"[84] That life-giving food might be stealing precious life from those who grow it. The burden of that responsibility is weighing on family farms like mine more now than ever before. So why do we do it? Perhaps you can blame it on our roots, our innate connection to the land, or the sheer belief that if we don't grow food, who will? That reliance and belief from consumers that food will always be available at the grocery store might not always be the case if farms keep disappearing from the landscape.

While bonfires and cornfields might romanticize the farming lifestyle to consumers, Kansas native Sarah Smarsh does a great job of highlighting the lack of social investments in rural areas in her book *Heartland: A Memoir of Working Hard and Being Broke in the Richest Country on Earth*. She writes, "The countryside is no more our nation's heart than are its cities, and rural people aren't more noble and dignified for their dirty work in fields. But to devalue, in our social investments, the people who tend crops and livestock, or to refer to their place as 'flyover country,' is to forget not just a country's foundation but its connection to the earth, to cycles of life scarcely witnessed and ill-understood in concrete landscapes."[85]

Better Mental Health in our Communities = Kindness, Compassion, and Love for Ourselves and Others

Just as I was beginning to write this last chapter, one of my best friends passed away suddenly. I felt challenged to my core about the message I was preaching on these pages while experiencing immense loss. It got me thinking that our mental wellness isn't just in the habits of how we live every day, it is also in the way we interact with those around us. Without our mental health, our bodies are just functional systems—a heart that beats blood through our veins and lungs that feed our organs. Living a life that nourishes our mental health means feeding those functional systems while practicing awareness, promoting gratitude, giving ourselves grace, and allowing ourselves to feel at every turn. Sometimes life hurts like hell, but we can't fully appreciate the good stuff without being handed the crap.

Each day is an opportunity to embrace what is in front of us, crap or not. This can be as simple as being more authentic with those around us or offering kindness and compassion. Can you recall a time when someone reached out to you when you needed it most? For me, it was one of my best friends that put her arm around my waist and held me up when my knees wanted to give out as I stood over an open casket and said goodbye to one of our friends. It was another friend who would pick up the phone when I needed her to, sometimes once a day and sometimes ten times a day. Those are the things that make us all vulnerable together; they are the things that connect us in our emotions.

Saskatchewan farmer Lesley Kelly experienced a similar moment from a stranger that she says will stay with her forever. Back in 2014, Lesley went to what she thought was a routine ultrasound appointment during her second pregnancy. In the midst of harvest on their farm, Lesley left her husband Matt at home to combine their crop and set off for the appointment alone. During the scan, the technician made a slight gasp, turned white, and left the room. "My heart sank," Kelly says. "I knew this wasn't good." A few moments later, the technician returned, this time alongside a doctor who started to explain that they found markers that showed the baby might have Down Syndrome and other health challenges. She was instructed to get more lab tests.

Lesley says she was in shock at the news while making her way to the lab. She took a number and sat down beside an elderly woman to wait for her turn to have blood drawn. She began to sob. Her heart was breaking and the fear of the information she was just told came out in long slow sobbing sounds and a river of tears. She says at that moment, the woman didn't say a word, she didn't ask what was wrong, she just grabbed her hand and held it tight while the tears streamed down her face. When the woman's number was called, she didn't get up, staying to hold Lesley's hand until it was Lesley's turn for the dreaded bloodwork that she feared would change the course of her family's life. When the test was done, Lesley returned to the waiting room, and the stranger who sat and comforted her was gone.

A few months later, Lesley and Matt Kelley's son Copeland arrived healthy. Lesley says, "Acts of kindness, love and hope, no matter how small or big are life changing and saving." That moment the kind woman sat with her, she says, "will stay with me for the rest of my life."

Lesley adds "I needed to feel someone comforting me, and that's what she did." The woman's actions, while small, are the kind of support we all need to collectively improve mental health in our communities.

CUE "HUMBLE AND KIND" BY TIM MCGRAW

While we need to show kindness and love to others, more importantly, we have to love ourselves, unconditionally, just as we are. We have an obligation to ourselves to nourish our mental wellness, but we owe it to everyone around us as well. We need to feel. And we need to allow others to feel as well. My view on mental wellness is that it will only get better as a society if we strive for it collectively while modeling it individually. When we can relinquish control, surrender to our emotions, validate them, and embrace whatever reality we are facing, only then can we truly be accountable for our own mental health.

A Princess without Purpose

Poor mental health isn't something that plagues only small towns and farming communities evening though high rates exist in this demographic. In March 2021, Meghan Markle was interviewed by Oprah about her mental health struggles while trying to assimilate into the royal family. A successful actress and businesswoman, Markle's ambitions were put aside after her marriage to Prince Harry in 2018, but it became clear that her new role and lack of independence did not suit her or her mental health. The responses I heard following that interview on CBS showed just how much our society has yet to learn when it comes to acknowledging mental health issues. As if her circumstance, or her wealth, had anything to do with her mental health problems, people criticized her vulnerabilities and questioned her emotions instead of validating them and showing compassion. It was heartbreaking to watch. It didn't matter how much money she had or how many people were on staff working for them. It didn't matter her title or that she married a prince. The thing she spoke about on television, in front of millions of people, was wanting to take her own life.[86] How brave she was! How vulnerable! Her mental health suffered, even under some of the best economic circumstances you could imagine in the world. This proved that mental illness does not discriminate. You can be a straight A student and struggle with depression, you can be an athlete and experience panic attacks, you can be a millionaire and still battle suicidal thoughts, and you can be a princess who simply wants independence. We are all allowed grace. Mental illness does not choose the poor, or the wealthy. It does not pick people living in the city, or in the country. And it has nothing to do with the colour of our skin, or where we grow up. Mental health affects us all, every day, under every circumstance, and sometimes despite our best efforts to stay on top of it.

Losing one of my best friends was, no doubt, devastating. But when I validate my emotions, and embrace reality, I am able to have realizations like finding gratitude: I am grateful for my kids and my husband and that I am still here every day able to be part of their lives. I am able to reach out and be vulnerable: consoling and supporting those around me with compassion while experiencing similar emotions of grief alongside them. I made sure, even this week, while moving through life (albeit very reluctantly) that I nourished my mental wellness by taking time to rest, making sure I moved my body, and by eating nutritious meals. It also meant making frozen chicken pot pies and frozen lasagna for a grieving family, because we do two things great in small towns: casseroles and rallying behind someone who needs help. Those small-town values are the ones I lean on to gain strength in my never-ending fight for mental health. That and music.

CUE "WHAT'S YOUR COUNTRY SONG" BY THOMAS RHETT

Songwriters are some of the best mental health experts. If you haven't already picked up on this from the music references in this book, know it now. Songwriters will always tell it like it is, advocating the same message I do—that we must feel it, all of it. Three chords and the truth might not fix your problems, but they might help you feel, hold your hand through heartbreak, help you kick up your heels when it is time for celebrations, and everything in between. Dierks Bentley cowrote a song alongside Ross Copperman, Ashley Gorley, and Jon Nite called *"Living"* and its lyrics might be some of the most honest I've heard to date.

"It's a beautiful world sometimes I don't see so clear." He goes on to sing, *"Some days you just get by, some days you're just alive, and some days you're living."*[87]

Spend more time living, but don't feel bad if some days you are just alive. Your self-worth doesn't change when your mental health fluctuates, and it also doesn't change when your productivity fluctuates. Nutrition, sleep, and exercise have been served up to us as ways to manage our weight, but what if your motivation becomes mental health? My guess is that if mental wellness is your motivation, you are more likely to take these tips and put them into practice. These are the most useful when used as preventative measures and mental health maintenance. If you are already in a dark place, please hear me when I say you deserve to get help now. If you have medication prescribed to you, make sure that you take it. You do not have to suffer.

In Canada, you can call the suicide prevention service at 1-833-456-4566 for help. In the United States you can call or text 988 for a crisis line. (This service is soon to be introduced in Canada as well.) The Kids Help Phone is another great one for young people. That number is 1-800-668-6868 or text CONNECT to 686868.

It is important and essential to find support if you are struggling. Professional counsellor Erica Hildebrand says mental health needs to be treated in the same way as other life-threatening diseases: "Think of someone who has cancer or a terminal illness. They rely on others to help them when they're going through treatment. Mental illness should be the same," she says. "You need people to help you when you're going through treatment." That treatment can look different for everyone. Only you can recognize what things make you feel better, and that's why treatment for each person can look very different.

A lot of mental injury can come from this one word: fear. Most of the mental injury from COVID was based in fear. We lived much of 2020 and 2021 living in fear of every sore throat, and every runny nose, and fear that we would make ourselves sick or make other people sick, fear that we aren't following the rules like we should or that we don't actually know the right rules. The fear was all-consuming and fear, I've discovered, does nothing for the joy in our life. That's because the best things in life are on the other side of fear.

While the virus took many lives around the world and I don't dispute or downplay that at all, I can't help but wonder: What damage did the fear leave behind? How many lives were lost? I have learned that the only way to counter the fear we feel in our lives is by choosing joy. (I can thank Rachel Hollis for that lesson too!) I have made choosing joy a lifelong mission because I know that when I am brave and choose joy, fear will diminish. I've heard some people say that choosing joy is not a remedy for depression. No, it is not. It is far more complicated than that. When you are deep in depression, you may not even have the capacity to feel joy at all. But it can grow again. I am proof of that. Sometimes I can choose joy and other days I have to fight damn hard to find it. As a good reminder, I only have to look as far as my birth certificate. While I might have been born an overthinker, Joy is still my middle name. That's not even a joke! My name at birth was Lewellyn Joy Laycock. That last name isn't a joke either, though I've heard them all so go ahead and have a good laugh. Maybe it was fate that my middle name is Joy. I never thought it suited me until recently. Now I can see that my middle name represents who I have become: A Fear Crusher and Joy-Seeker. It is why I decided to take up the opportunity to go skydiving in my twenties, why I decided to leave my media career to farm alongside my husband, why I started running races in my thirties, and also why I decided to write this book as I approach my forties. Those things were laced with fear. I acknowledged the fear, but I chose to do them in pursuit of joy. I've discovered my mental health will never flourish when I live in fear, but it will when I fight for joy.

Because of my own struggles, whenever my kids are having a bad day, I immediately want to fix it for them. I can't, and that isn't my job as a parent either. My job, as a parent, and my purpose with this book, is the same for you as for my children: to teach the tools required to look after your own mental health. I read a statistic lately we can't ignore: 4.6 million children called Kids Help Phone in 2020. In contrast, 1.9 million called in 2019.[88] Some people might read this statistic and be devastated at the fact that kids have been under extreme mental injury. I agree they were under immense mental injury in 2020. However, I look at this statistic with such pride. I can see that we are normalizing the conversation around mental health and that kids feel comfortable enough to get help, wherever they can find it. What a blessing! No one should ever feel guilt about asking for help or having to battle mental illness alone. We all deserve to have a helping hand when we need it, especially our kids.

Keep Feeling, and Keep Talking

CUE "PEOPLE DON'T TALK ABOUT" BY THE REKLAWS

The 4-H slogan got it right (if you are a prairie kid you will get the reference here): "You learn to do by doing." When we don't talk about the hard stuff, it does not serve our mental health. So get comfortable being uncomfortable. We can work out, eat all our vegetables, and get sleep, but if we don't talk about the stuff going on in our heart and our head, we are still going be mentally unwell. (It is also really hard for joy to get through a thick layer of exhaustion I've found.)

My husband and I recently watched a movie called *A Beautiful Day in the Neighbourhood* that had Tom Hanks playing the role of Mr. Rogers. The movie portrayed how the TV star lived his life and the lessons he tried to teach kids, as well as the adults who were around him. Many of these lessons are based in psychology. Tom Hanks' character offered advice to a family who is watching their father die and finding it hard to talk about death. "Death is something many of us are uncomfortable speaking about. But to die is to be human. And anything human is mentionable. Anything mentionable is manageable."[89] I love the simplicity in this message. Not just death, but if it is a part of life, isn't it worth talking about? We forget how basic it can be to honour our mental health. When we understand feelings of guilt, fear, or pain might be a temporary outcome, we can see the reward that comes with talking about things with vulnerability, authenticity and honesty even and especially if they make us uncomfortable. We have an obligation to foster connection and improve mental health together: in our health care, in our schools, in our families, and in our communities. If a child is taught that certain topics are off the table to discuss, it simply teaches them to deal with it alone. We can't pay for hurtful silence with our health, or our lives. Sometimes we need to stand beside each other, sometimes we need to lean on each other, other times we need to hold each other up from crumbling to the floor or sometimes we need to crumble alongside each other.

Mental health can be supported without actually talking about mental health too. For example, the mental health of farmers might improve by something as simple as risk management, succession planning, and budgeting. Showing we care about others can be as simple as making eye contact, offering a smile or a wave. If you can't find the words, start with small actions. And if you want to start talking about your feelings, you must start by learning what is going in your body first. Self-awareness is key. I was able to walk down the path to healing only when I listened to my body the same way I listened to music.

I'll Keep Healing Loudly, So Others Won't Die Quietly

CUE UP "BETTER THAN WE FOUND IT" BY MAREN MORRIS

Female singer/songwriter Maren Morris wrote "Better Than We Found It" alongside Jessie Jo Dillon, Jimmy Robbins, and Laura Veltz. It speaks about modelling change for others. Morris sings "Who's gonna care if I don't? Who's gonna change if I won't?"[90] I believe this song was written for the Black Lives Matter movement, which is another important change we are seeing in the world, but I think the lyrics and this movement illustrate that we always have a choice to either do nothing or speak up when we have the chance. My journey has left me thinking that I have the ability to teach others about mental wellness, so why would I sit quietly? I'm healing loudly now. I could have taken my own life at the age of twelve. I could have chosen fear. But fear did not win. Joy did. My saving didn't happen in a church pew that day. I didn't pray it away. My healing happened through life's experiences: when I changed careers, trading cameras for canola; it happened when I became a mom and gave up a piece of myself to my kids then fought to get my sense of self back; and it happened when I started speaking out about my mental health journey. Music is like life, and I'm determined to play it loud.

I've discovered that life isn't about being happy all the time. I've discovered I don't have to be perfect either. Once I take the pressure off with those two realizations, life becomes about the experiences—the good times, bad times, the mundane everyday moments, and everything in between. Without adversity, we cannot experience resilience. Without sadness, pain, and hurt, there is no ability to feel joy. We must feel it all.

For me, being strong in my small town used to mean putting on a brave face and hiding my emotions to protect myself and others. But strength isn't our capacity to handle stress, trauma, neglect, or abuse. I also thought that being strong meant hiding my vulnerabilities, which in fact, turns out to be my strengths. Small town strong has taken on new meaning for me. It means showing up with all my vulner-abilities. It means making space to hold my own emotions and the emotions of others around me. We all need compassion. We all deserve some grace. I'm giving new meaning to small-town strong, modeling what real mental wellness looks like: being real, raw, and vulnerable, and showing compassion and grace when needed. Allowing myself to feel, free of guilt has brought me so much wisdom. Do you know what else helps us feel? Crying. Crying is one of the most beautiful things you can do, yet haven't we been taught to fight the urge when it comes? Stop fighting it. Crying is one of the most therapeutic activities there are. It activates the parasympathetic nervous system and lowers cortisol levels. There is no shame in it, and you don't have to justify it either. Let yourself cry. It is your body trying to self regulate. Let it do its job.

When I look back at my past, I often think about how much I might have missed out on because of my depression or anxiety, but if I erase my emotions and experiences from the past, I also erase the wisdom of my present. I don't think I've recovered from my depression or anxiety per se, because mental health is something that we must manage daily. No one is immune to struggling with mental health. No one. Do I still have bad days? Hell ya! I just don't make those bad days make me feel like a bad person or make me believe that I have a bad life. Sometimes a bad day is just that—a bad day. I used to let those things make me believe that I was broken, but I have realized that I was never broken. I wasn't broken when I suffered suicidal thoughts as a child. I wasn't broken when I suffered anxiety as a young mother, Taneal wasn't broken when she suffered postpartum depression, and Kristyn wasn't broken when she was grieving the loss of her husband either. We weren't broken, we were human. The kind of humans that have felt so deeply that is impossible not to reach out a hand to others when they need it, because we are embracing the highly empathetic and compassionate beings that we are, through the life experiences we were handed. We are the ones that will stand up alongside others who are walking through big emotions. The ones who will stand up for mental health each step of the way.

Learning how to tune into my body and listen to what I need to stay well has taken time. That self-awareness has become a crucial component to improving my mental health and comes with an understanding that my feelings aren't problems that need to be fixed or ignored. They are simply messages from my body telling me how I'm doing and what I need. Regulating my nervous system really means listening to my body carefully each day like listening to a song that quickly changes key and diverts into a bridge away from its original melody.

After a long day of work in the summer, I can recognize when I need to rest and recharge. Sometimes, I'll recharge by going for a kayak or a paddle board on a lake just a couple of miles from our home. My honey hole is a little piece of heaven on the west side of a 140-acre field where I have a little swing to sit and take in the prairie's breathtaking beauty. During the summer months, I often have a feeling that I live in one of the most beautiful places on Earth. When I drive down these roads and pass quarters of land that were cleared over a century ago at the hand of some of the first farmers in this area, I am assured that the seasons will always be changing, as will the hands of the people who tend to this land, but the land is the constant here. Somehow, I have put to rest the notion that I didn't belong on the farm. I am meant to be here. I can feel it. Nothing but the land is permanent. Not the trees in the shelterbelt surrounding our yard, not my chickens pecking the ground. Not a feeling. Not a bad day or a good day. Not me. It is all fleeting. I also have the feeling that the farm isn't stealing life from me, but rather challenging me to muster all that I have within me while I'm here, just like the leaves transforming before winter. Sharing my story is vital for the survival of our industry, and the farm families dedicating their lives to it. Will my next project be song writing? Maybe. In the meantime, I know my feet are rooted right where they are meant to be.

CUE "THIS AIN'T HEAVEN" BY ERIN KINSEY

I know that I can be uncomfortable when winter hits, assured that when spring arrives, I will hear the croak of the frogs out my window when I lie down to go to sleep, and hear the rain drops on our tin roof when the summer rains arrive. I won't just hear them, I will feel them like a stranger reaching out to hold my hand, reassuring me that in each season I have exactly what I need inside myself to continue growing here. I will no longer live in survival mode, instead I will start simply living. I may have been raised in a culture of hard work, and chose a profession that breeds burnout, but I am aware that my self-worth isn't tied to my productivity, my emotions don't make me weak, and that I deserve unconditional love just as I am and especially from myself, in any season. Wherever life leads you, and whatever life throws at you, understand that you also deserve that. We all deserve that, and none of us are broken.

CUE UP "GOOD TO BE ALIVE" BY MEGHAN TRAINER

You better crank this one up and do some dancing!

A plea to my readers: If you enjoyed this book, please share a review on social media. Make sure to tag me in it and use the hashtag #Rooted. Other ways you can help get this important message into the world is by recommending it to a friend, by leaving a review on Goodreads or Amazon, or by asking your local bookstore or library to stock it. Those are the best ways to support authors like myself, as well as change the culture around mental health. I appreciate you taking the time to read this book. *Take care of you always.*

ACKNOWLEDGMENTS

First off, I want to thank my husband James who always encouraged me to write this book, years before I actually sat down to do it. He has always believed in my ability to write, in a meaningful way, even before I did. He encouraged me to write about my story despite being a very private person. My ability to get raw and real is, no doubt, because of his encouragement and the encouragement of so many of my friends who sometimes didn't understand my battle with mental illness or my reasons behind writing this book, but loved me through it anyways. That is real unconditional love and for that, I am forever grateful.

I want to thank my kids, who were too young to understand the importance of the book I was writing but knew loving their mom meant standing behind whatever it was she was doing in the office early in the mornings, late at night, on the weekends, while they were at school, and even the editing that overflowed into their Christmas break and summer holidays. Ava, you are wise beyond your years. You are armed with the emotional intelligence I wish I had at your age. I have no doubt that the beauty and fire in your soul will change the world. You once told me that maybe one day I would win the Nellie McClung Foundation's trailblazer award for writing this book. The fact that you know about that award, created to honour a prairie woman who brought about change in society, tells me I've raised you right (and that you also had Mr. Baskerville as a teacher). Accolades are lovely, but if I never win an award for this book, I will not be phased at all because you and Lane are my greatest achievements and always will be. Lane, you are a firecracker, and with your perseverance, energy, and passion, I know you are armed with the skills to do anything and a heart big enough to know the reasons why.

Megan Shipp, thank you for being my biggest teacher, role model, and cheerleader in life. You have always been one step ahead of me and paved the way for me. Being a trailblazer yourself, especially in a small town, is never easy. Don't ever stop being so brave. Also, I expect you to trim the branches on this bush trail for me and many other women for many more years to come, so keep those trimmers handy!

I have to thank Rachel Hollis and her entire community of women who made me truly believe that I was made for more. Their support and commitment to lift up other women has been immeasurable. Thank you for teaching me to rise.

Brené Brown, I have to thank you for all of the teachings you have put out into the world that have been parallel to my beliefs. They are making the world a better place, and for that, I am forever grateful.

A huge thank you goes out to everyone who contributed to this book: Dr. Wendy Davis, Dr. Erica Hildebrand, Dr. James Rae, Megan Shipp, Lesley Kelly, and especially Taneal Semeniuk and Kristyn Eftoda. Your vulnerability and resilience will truly change the lives of many people who will read this. Making mental wellness a priority is easy to do when there are people like you to show us how.

Thank you to my mom Veronica who was my advocate, my role model, and a kick-ass female farmer who likes to say bad words at appropriate and justified times. You rock. Keep taking breaks from the farm. You deserve it. Dad, thanks for working so hard for us. I know it wasn't easy.

Thank you to my sister Brandy for moving to Angusville. I will come to you wherever you move, but I love that you moved closer to me. We need each other and always will. You have always had my back and I will always have yours.

Thank you to Jill Rothenberg whose knowledge and expertise as an editor made this book what it is. Our passion for the written word, running, and farm boys (or cowboys in your case) has connected us on a level I never expected, but I am so grateful for. Working alongside you has been such a pleasure.

Thank you to Jessica Schnieder at Your Story Media for producing my audio book over your Christmas break and in between parenting. You are the kind of entrepreneur I am proud to work with.

Thank you to Alicia Grassinger, our small-town librarian, who I have kept busy for many days searching for books.

Someone once told me to find the thing that makes you lose track of time. I've lost track of a good chunk of the last two and a half years, but it has been so worth it.

While I wrote this book, I continually pictured the audience that would be reading it, especially my girlfriends: Megan, Kalen, Kathy, Sheri, Carly, Jenn, Christa, Shawna, and Karen. What I didn't know was that Karen wouldn't get enough time to read it before passing away. Thank you to these ladies and all the people who will read this book and continue to live the messages within it. You are my mental health warriors. Thank you. I am forever grateful for you all.

Auntie Jean you are incredible. You have been such an incredible role model for me. I am rooted here because of the help and guidance you and Uncle John have offered us over the years. Thank you.

Susan, Chery, and Shelby: what can I say, except that I think Baba Melnyk would be proud of the work we all do on this farm and may we honour her legacy in everything we do here. She would be so proud.

♫ PLAYLIST ♫

"A Song for Everything," by Maren Morris

"Jolene," by Dolly Parton

"Hard Workin' Man," by Brooks and Dunn

"Where Corn Don't Grow," by Travis Tritt

"Strawberry Wine," by Deanna Carter

"The House That Built Me," by Miranda Lambert

"When You Call My Name," by Paul Brandt

"Fight Song," by Rachel Platten

"Wide Open Spaces," by The Chicks

"Easy on Me," by Adele

"Farmer," by Lee Brice

"How Can I Help You to Say Goodbye," by Patty Loveless

"Sit Still, Look Pretty," by Daya

"Crazy Bitch," by Buckcherry

"Smoke Break," by Carrie Underwood

"Run," by OneRepublic

"Run," by Lauren Alaina

"Kick off Your Boots," by Hawg Wylde

"Fenceposts," by Cody Johnson

"Chicken Fried," by Zac Brown Band

"Rollin' (The Ballad of Big & Rich)," by Big & Rich

"I Should Probably Go to Bed," by Dan + Shay

"Mother's Daughter," by Miley Cyrus

"Let's Talk About Sex," by Salt-N-Pepa

"Small Towns and Big Dreams," by Paul Brandt

"Anywhere with You," by Jake Owen

"Never Til Now," by Ashley Cooke, Brett Young

"I Love Myself Today," by Bif Naked

"Rise Up," by Andra Day

"Girl," by Maren Morris

"Next to You, Next to Me," by Shenandoah

"Famous in a Small Town," by Miranda Lambert

"Whiskey Glasses," by Morgan Wallen

"Sad Girls Do Sad Things," by Priscilla Block

"Mapdot," by Jess Moskaluke

"Small Town Small," by Jason Aldean

"Ironic," by Alanis Morissette

"abcdefu," by GAYLE

"The Truck Got Stuck," by Corb Lund

"Shake It Off," by Taylor Swift

"London Rain," by Heather Nova

"Why Haven't I Heard from You," by Reba McEntire

"I Try to Think About Elvis," by Patty Loveless

"In My Veins," by Lauren Alaina

"Confident," by Demi Lovato

"I'm Not for Everyone," by Brothers Osborne

"Doubt Me Now," by Cody Johnson

"The Race Is On," by Sawyer Brown

"Drowning," by Chris Young

"The Climb," by Miley Cyrus

"Where I'm From," by The Reklaws

"Humble and Kind," by Tim McGraw

"What's Your Country Song," by Thomas Rhett

"Living," by Dierks Bentley

"People Don't Talk About," by the Reklaws

"Better than We Found It," by Maren Morris

"This Ain't Heaven," by Erin Kinsey

"Good to Be Alive," by Meghan Trainer

⬘ RECOMMENDED READS ⬘

Focus on the 90%: One Simple Tool to Change the Way You View Your Life, by Darci Lang

Girl, Stop Apologizing: A Shame-Free Plan for Embracing and Achieving Your Goals, by Rachel Hollis

Girl, Wash Your Face: Stop Believing the Lies About Who You Are So You Can Become Who You Were Meant to Be, by Rachel Hollis

Good Morning, I Love You: Mindfulness and Self-Compassion Practices to Rewire Your Brain for Calm, Clarity, and Joy, by Shauna Shapiro

Happiness In Your Life series, by Doe Zantamata

Healthy Healing, by Michelle Steinke-Baumgard

Heartland: A Memoir of Working Hard and Being Broke in the Richest Country on Earth, by Sarah Smarsh

Hormone Repair Manual, by Dr. Lara Briden

It's OK that You're Not OK, by Megan Devine

Just One Thing, by Rick Hanson

Kids These Days, by Dr. Jody Carrington

Resilient: How to Grow an Unshakable Core of Calm, Strength, and Happiness by Rick Hanson

Swing, by Ashleigh Renard

Teachers These Days, by Dr. Jody Carrington

The 5 Love Languages, by Gary Chapman

The 7 Habits of Highly Effective People: Restoring the Character Ethic, by Stephen Covey

The Gifts of Imperfection, by Brené Brown What Makes Olga Run? The Mystery of the 90-Something Track Star and What She Can Teach Us About Living Longer, Happier Lives, by Bruce Grierson

When the Body Says No, by Gabor Maté

ENDNOTES

1   "A Song for Everything," Spotify, track 4 on Maren Morris, Girl, Sony Music Entertainment, 2019.

2   Alison Kennedy, Julie Cerel, Athena Kheibari, Stuart Leske, and James Watts, "A Comparison of Farming- and Non-Farming-Related Suicides from the United States' National Violent Deaths Reporting System, 2003–2016," *Suicide and Life-Threatening Behavior 51*, no. 3 (January 2021), https://doi.org/10.1111/sltb.12725.

3   Andria Jones-Bitton et al., "Stress, Anxiety, Depression, and Resilience in Canadian Farmers," *Social Psychiatry and Psychiatric Epidemiology 55*, (2020). https://doi.org/10.1007/s00127-019-01738-2.

4   Dale Kawashima, "Lainey Wilson Talks About Her Hit "Things A Man Oughta Know", Her Album *Sayin' What I'm Thinkin'*, And Writing Her Songs" Songwriter Universe, June 14, 2021.

5   "When You Call My Name," Spotify, track 7 on Paul Brandt, *Small Towns and Big Dreams*, Brand-T Records, 2001.

6   Anjel Vahration et al., "Symptoms of Anxiety or Depressive Disorder and Use of Mental Health Care Among Adults During the COVID-19 Pandemic – United States, August 2020-February 2021." MMWR 70, (2021): 490-494, http://dx.doi.org/10.15585/mmwr.mm7013e2.

7   Gregory Jaynes, "U.S. Farmers Said to Face Worse Year Since1930s," *The New York Times*, March 28, 1982, 1.

8   "Mental Illness–Symptoms and Causes," Mayo Clinic, June 8, 2019, https://www.mayoclinic.org/diseases-conditions/mental-illness/symptoms-causes/syc-20374968#:~:text=Mental%20illness%2C%20also%20called%20mental,eating%20disorders%20and%20addictive%20behaviors.

9   *Fast Facts about Mental Health and Mental Illness*. Canadian Mental Health Association website. July 19, 2021. www.cmha.ca

10   Gabor Maté, *When the Body Says No*, (Toronto: Random House Canada, 2003), 23.

11   Julie Tseng and Jordan Poppenk, "Brain Meta-State Transitions Demarcate Thoughts Across Task Contexts Exposing the Mental Noise of Trait Neuroticism." Nature Communications 11, no. 3480 (2020), https://doi.org/10.1038/s41467-020-17255-9.

12   Darci Lang, *Focus on the 90%: One Simple Tool to Change the Way You View Your Life*, (X-L Enterprises Inc., 2010).

13   Shauna Shapiro, Good Morning, I Love You: Mindfulness and Self-Compassion Practices to Rewire Your Brain for Calm, Clarity, and Joy. (Boulder: Sounds True, 2020).

14   Matthew A. Killingsworth and Daniel T. Gilbert, "A Wandering Mind Is an Unhappy Mind," *Science* 330, (2010), https://www.science.org/doi/abs/10.1126/science.1192439.

15   "Mindfulness Defined. What Is Mindfulness?" *Greater Good Magazine*. https://greatergood.berkeley.edu/topic/mindfulness/definition#:~:text=Mindfulness%20means%20maintaining%20a%20moment,through%20a%20gentle%2C%20nurturing%20lens.

16   Dr. Erica Hildebrand, Interview with Professional Counsellor, e-mail interview with the author, April 6, 2021.

17   "Depression and Other Common Mental Disorders: Global Health Estimates by the World Health Organization," Geneva: World Health Organization, (2017) http://apps.who.int/iris/bitstream/handle/10665/254610/WHO-MSD-MER-2017.2-eng.f;jsessionid=F5BEBC48140F133E8D3E4EF87D23FBE2?sequence=1.

18   Sandra Lopez-Leon et al., "More than 50 Long-Term Effects of COVID-19: A Systematic Review and Meta-Analysis," *Scientific Reports* 11, (August 2021), https://www.nature.com/articles/s41598-021-95565-8#citeas.

19   Yomi Akinpelu, *Blow the Cap off Your Capability: Be Unstoppable*, (Kent: Pneuma Springs Publishing, 2020), 237.

20   Stephen R. Covey, *The 7 Habits of Highly Effective People*, (New York: Free Press, 2004) 161.

21   Amanda Williams, "Five Exercises That Help Manage Anxiety–And One You Might Want to Avoid," Fitbit, February 2, 2018. https://blog.fitbit.com/exercises-to-manage-anxiety/.

22   Martina Kanning and Wolfgang Schlicht, "Be Active and Become Happy: An Ecological Momentary Assessment of Physical Activity and Mood," *Journal of Sport and Exercise Psychology* 32, 2 (April 2010): 253–61, doi: 10.1123/jsep.32.2.253.

23   "Moving Toward a Better Normal: ParticipACTION Report Card on Physical Activity for Adults, 2021" ParticipACTION, November 30, 2021, https://participaction.cdn.prismic.io/participaction/e98e050d-90a2-43bd-a49d-e7c288071725_2021-ParticipACTION-Report-Card-on-Physical-Activity-for-Adults.pdf.

24   "Sour Mood Getting You Down? Get Back to Nature," Harvard Health Publishing: Harvard Medical School, March 30, 2021, https://www.health.harvard.edu/mind-and-mood/sour-mood-getting-you-down-get-back-to-nature.

25   For a list of helpful tips for boundaries on the farm, visit The Do More Agriculture Foundation's website: www.domore.ag.

26   Kaida Ning et al., "Association of Relative Brain Age with Tobacco Smoking, Alcohol Consumption, and Genetic Variants," *Scientific Reports* 10, (January 2020) https://doi.org/10.1038/s41598-019-56089-4.

27   Doe Zantamata, *Quotes About Living: Quotes from the Happiness in Your Life Book Series*. (Scotts Valley: CreateSpace, 2014), 80.

28   Christian Benedict et al., "Acute Sleep Deprivation Enhances the Brain's Response to Hedonic Food Stimuli: An fMRI Study," *The Journal of Clinical Endocrinology and Metabolism* 97, no. 3, (March 2012): E443–E447, accessed March 22, 2022, https://doi.org/10.1210/jc.2011-2759.

29   Anika Knüppel et al., "Sugar Intake from Sweet Food and Beverages, Common Mental Disorder and Depression: Prospective Findings from the Whitehall II Study," *Scientific Reports* 7, (July 2017), https://doi.org/10.1038/s41598-017-05649-7.

30   G. Grases et al., "Possible Relation Between Consumption of Different Food Groups and Depression," BMC *Psychology* 7, (2019), https://doi.org/10.1186/s40359-019-0292-1.

31   Megan Shipp, Healthy Eating Coach Interview, in discussion with the author, July 21, 2021.

32   Kristen E. D'Anci et al., "Voluntary Dehydration and Cognitive Performance in Trained College Athletes," *Perceptual and Motor Skills* 109, no. 1 (August 2009): 251–69. https://doi.org/10.2466/pms.109.1.251-269.

33   Lawrence E. Armstrong et al. "Mild Dehydration Affects Mood in Healthy Young Women," *The Journal of Nutrition* 142, no. 2 (February 2012): 382–d388, https://doi.org/10.3945/jn.111.142000.

34   Martha Clare Morris et al., "Nutrients and Bioactives in Green Leafy Vegetables and Cognitive Decline: Prospective Study," *Neurology* 90 (January 2018): e214-e222. doi: 10.1212/WNL.0000000000004815.

35   Jane Clatworthy, Joe Hinds, and Paul M. Camic, "Gardening as a Mental Health Intervention: A Review," *Mental Health Review Journal*, (2013), https://www.emerald.com/insight/content/doi/10.1108/MHRJ-02-2013-0007/full/html.

36   R. Mocking et al., "Meta-Analysis and Meta-Regression of Omega-3 Polyunsaturated Fatty Acid Supplementation for Major Depressive Disorder," *Translational Psychiatry* 6, (2016), https://doi.org/10.1038/tp.2016.29.

37   S.V. Ramesh et al., "Dietary Prospects of Coconut Oil for the Prevention and Treatment of Alzheimer's Disease (AD): A Review of Recent evidences," *Trends in Food Science & Technology* 112, (2021): 201–211, https://www.sciencedirect.com/science/article/abs/pii/S0924224421002387

38   Bettina Moritz et al., "The Role of Vitamin C in Stress-Related Disorders," *The Journal of Nutritional Biochemistry* 85, (November 2020) https://www.sciencedirect.com/science/article/pii/S0955286320304915.

39   Maureen M. Leonard et al., "Celiac Disease and Nonceliac Gluten Sensitivity: A Review," JAMA, (August 2017): 647–656. https://jamanetwork.com/journals/jama/article-abstract/2648637.

40   Amber Pariona, "What Are the World's Most Important Staple Foods?" WorldAtlas, June 7, 2019. https://www.worldatlas.com/articles/most-important-staple-foods-in-the-world.html#:~:text=Wheat%20is%20typically%20dried%20and,calorie%20intake%20comes%20from%20wheat

41   John R. Kelly et al., "Transferring the Blues: Depression-Associated Gut Microbiota Induces Neurobehavioural Changes in the Rat," *Journal of Psychiatric Research* 82, (November 2016):109–118 https://www.sciencedirect.com/science/article/abs/pii/S0022395616301571.

42   "Will the CICO Diet Help You Lose Weight," video, 7:57, YouTube, posted by Jillian Michaels, January 12, 2021. https://www.youtube.com/watch?v=-PsZFvLlwoE.

43   Dr. Wendy Davis, Naturopath Interview, in discussion with the author, December 16, 2020.

44   Alexander Panossian and Georg Wikman, "Effects of Adaptogens on the Central Nervous System and the Molecular Mechanisms Associated with Their Stress—Protective Activity," Pharmaceuticals 3, no. 1, (2010): 188–224. https://www.mdpi.com/1424-8247/3/1/188.

45   Lionel Noah et al., "Effect of Vitamin B6 Supplementation, in Combination with Magnesium, on Severe Stress and Magnesium Status: Secondary Analysis from an RCT," The Proceedings of the Nutrition Society 79, no. OCE2 (2020): E491, doi:10.1017/S0029665120004395.

46   Rebecca Costello et al., "Perspective: The Case for an Evidence-Based Reference Interval for Serum Magnesium: The Time Has Come," Advances in Nutrition: An International Review Journal 7, (November 2016): 977–993, https://www.ncbi.nlm.nih.gov/pmc/articles/PMC5105038/.

47   Ann Wigmore, The Hippocrates Diet and Health Program: A Natural Diet and Health Program for Weight Control, Disease Prevention, and Life Extension, (New York: Avery, 1983) 9.

48   Abraham H. Maslow, "A Theory of Human Motivation," Psychological Review 50, no. 4 (1943): 370–396, https://psycnet.apa.org/doiLanding?doi=10.1037%2Fh0054346.

49   Andre Sólo, "How to Explain High Sensitivity to People Who Don't 'Get' It," Highly Sensitive Refuge, August 15, 2018, https://highlysensitiverefuge.com/explain-high-sensitivity/.

50   Dr. James Rae, Rural Doctor Interview, in discussion with the author, February 15, 2021.

51   Dave Monson, "I made a new rule: Never trust how you feel about your entire life past 9pm," Twitter user @drewmonson7, January 6, 2022.

52   Yellowstone, season 3, episode 3, "An Acceptable Surrender," directed by Taylor Sheridan, written by Taylor Sheridan and John Linson, aired July 5, 2020, on Paramount Network.

53   Andria Jones-Bitton, "Stress, Anxiety, Depression, and Resilience in Canadian Farmers," Social Psychiatry and Psychiatric Epidemiology 55, (2020), https://doi.org/10.1007/s00127-019-01738-2

54   Sarah Smarsh, Heartland: A Memoir of Working Hard and Being Broke in the Richest Country on Earth, (New York; Scribner, 2018), 251.

55   A. Pawlowski, "These Are the States with the Highest and Lowest Life Expectancy," Today, February 15, 2022, https://www.today.com/health/health/life-expectancy-highest-hawaii-california-rcna16133.

56   Jenn Hardy (@drjennhardy), "Affordable Self Care: Set more realistic expectations about how long things take to get done," Instagram photo, August 10, 2021.

57   "Chronic Stress Puts Your Health at Risk," Mayo Clinic, June 8, 2021, https://www.mayoclinic.org/healthy-lifestyle/stress-management/in-depth/stress/art-20046037.

58   Doe Zantamata, *Quotes About Living: Quotes from the Happiness in Your Life Book Series,* (CreateSpace, 2014), 82.

59   Taneal Semeniuk, Overcoming Post Partum Depression Interview, in discussion with the author, January 11, 2021.

60   Maté, *When the Body Says No,* 27.

61   James C. Fleet et al., "Vitamin D and Cancer: A Review of Molecular Mechanisms," *Biochemical Journal 441,* no. 1 (January 2012): 61–76, https://doi.org/10.1042/BJ20110744

62   Brené Brown, *The Gifts of Imperfection: Let Go of Who You Think You're Supposed to Be and Embrace Who You Are,* (Center City: Hazelden Publishing, 2010) 19.

63   Ashleigh Renard, Marriage Interview with author of Swing, in discussion with the author, March 9, 2021.

64   Ashleigh Renard, *Swing,* (Galway: MW Books, 2021), 287.

65   Brown, *The Gifts of Imperfection,* 47.

66   Jason Medows, "ASOM – Ep 124 – Elaine Froese – Farm Family Coach – Part 1" February 16, 2022, in *Ag State of Mind,* podcast, 38:23, https://open.spotify.com/episode/37hDhxqkvoAHOIWrLiyJUU.

67   "How Alcohol Actually Increases Stress Levels Rather Than Relaxing You," video, 6:57, YouTube, posted by Huberman Lab Clips, January 2, 2023. https://www.youtube.com/watch?v=4xU5yIH_P9I

68   Farm Management Canada, *Healthy Minds, Healthy Farms, Exploring the connection between Mental Health and Farm Business Management,* May 2020. https://fmc-gac.com/wp-content/uploads/2020/07/finalreport.pdf.

69   Dr. James Rae, Rural Doctor Interview, in discussion with the author, February 15, 2021.

70   Kendra Cherry, "What Is Neuroplasticity?" Verywell Mind, last modified September 19, 2022. https://www.verywellmind.com/what-is-brain-plasticity-2794886#:~:text=Neuroplasticity%2C%20also%20known%20as%20brain,as%20a%20result%20of%20experience.

71   James Redfield, *The Celestine Prophecy,* (New York: Grand Central Publishing, 2008). The Interpersonal Ethic: Part 6 Healing Your Relationships.

72   Covey, *The 7 Habits of Highly Effective People,* 72.

73   Britta K. Hölzel, et al., "How Does Mindfulness Meditation Work? Proposing Mechanisms of Action From a Conceptual and Neural Perspective," *Perspectives on Psychological Science 6,* no. 6 (November 2011): 537–559, doi:10.1177/1745691611419671.

74   Jenn Hardy (@drjennhardy), "It's hard to tune into your intuitive voice if you never let yourself slow down enough to actually hear it," Instagram photo, August 22, 2021, https://www.instagram.com/p/CS5eEcnMTAl/?igshid=YmMyMTA2M2Y= .

75   *Colour Oxford English Dictionary*, (Oxford: Oxford University Press, 2011), 754.

76   Bruce Grierson, *What Makes Olga Run? The Mystery of the 90-Something Track Star and What She Can Teach Us About Living Longer, Happier Lives*, (New York: Henry Holt & Company., 2014).

77   Rachel Hollis, *Girl, Stop Apologizing: A Shame-Free Plan for Embracing and Achieving Your Goals*, (New York: HarperCollins Leadership, 2019), 94.

78   Kristyn Eftoda, Overcoming Grief Interview, in discussion with the author, February 22, 2021.

79   Kate Allsopp, "Heterogeneity in Psychiatric Diagnostic Classification," *Psychiatry Research 279*, (July 2019): 15-22, doi:10.1016/j.psychres.2019.07.005.

80   University of Liverpool, "Psychiatric Diagnosis 'Scientifically Meaningless,'" ScienceDaily, July 8, 2019, https://www.sciencedaily.com/releases/2019/07/190708131152.htm.

81   "Canada's 2021 Census of Agriculture: A story about the transformation of the agriculture industry and adaptiveness of Canadian farmers," Statistics Canada, May 11, 2021,

82   "Ag and Food Sectors and the Economy," Economic Research Service USDA, last modified February 24, 2022,

83   *Fast Facts About Agriculture & Food*, American Farm Bureau website, 2021.

84   "Where I'm From," Spotify, track 8 on The Reklaws, *Sophomore Slump*, Universal Music Canada, 2020.

85   Smarsh, *Heartland: A Memoir of Working Hard and Being Broke in the Richest Country on Earth*, 122.

86   *Oprah with Meghan and Harry: A CBS Primetime Special*, CBS, March 7, 2021.

87   "Living," Spotify, track on 3 Dierks Bentley, *The Mountain*, Capitol Nashville, 2018

88   "Kids Help Phone Celebrates 20th Anniversary with Fundraiser," Kids Help Phone, May 13, 2021. https://kidshelpphone.ca/publications/kids-help-phone-celebrates-20th-anniversary-with-fundraiser.

89   Marielle Heller, dir., *A Beautiful Day in the Neighborhood*, (Culver City: TriStar Pictures, November 22, 2019).

90   "Better than We Found It," Spotify, single, Maren Morris, Sony Music Entertainment, 2020.